Practice Questions

1. A seven-month-old baby shows decreased abduction of his left leg, thigh fold asymmetry, and disparity of leg lengths. Choose the test maneuver or sign to evaluate the baby for developmental hip dysplasia:
   a. Barlow maneuver
   b. Ortolani test
   c. Allis' sign
   d. Adam's forward bend test

2. To meet Medicare's coverage requirements, the Nurse Practitioner's services must be:
   a. Provided subject to state restrictions and supervision requirements
   b. Provided under direct supervision
   c. Provided in a rural health clinic (RHC) or federally qualified health center (FQHC)
   d. Billed through a physician-directed clinic, health agency, or hospital

3. Angiotensin-converting enzyme (ACE) inhibitors are contraindicated for patients with:
   a. Hypertension
   b. Diabetes mellitus
   c. Heart failure
   d. Renal failure

4. Patient-focused goal setting should be:
   a. Mandated and controlled by the clinician
   b. Reasonable, measurable, and achievable
   c. Simple
   d. Long-term rather than short-term

5. Your 20-year-old male patient has epistaxis. You observe him bleeding from both posterior nares and swallowing, so you apply topical vasoconstrictors and pack his nostrils. After 30 minutes, his bleeding stops. Choose the follow-up blood tests, if any:
   a. No blood test is necessary for a simple nosebleed
   b. Hematocrit and hemoglobin to determine his blood loss
   c. Coagulation panel
   d. Complete blood count

6. Your 86-year-old patient has end-stage cardiac disease. Her doctor wrote a Do-Not-Resuscitate order in her chart. In her advance directive, your patient explicitly declined life-prolonging procedures. However, when your patient arrests, her daughter demands the nurses perform CPR. The staff should:
    a. Proceed with CPR, as the patient can no longer make her own decisions
    b. Proceed with CPR while calling the patient's physician to verify the DNR order
    c. Contact the Ethics Committee for guidance
    d. Advise her daughter that CPR must be withheld, in accordance with her mother's wishes

7. When wearing a Holter monitor, the patient should:
    a. Refrain from taking cardiac medications
    b. Restrict activities
    c. Maintain an activity diary
    d. Turn it off during the night

8. Your 70-year-old female patient has a gallop rhythm. You detected S3 occurring after S2 through auscultation, with your patient lying on her left side. This may be indicative of:
    a. Aortic stenosis
    b. Mitral stenosis
    c. Pericarditis
    d. Heart failure or left ventricular failure

9. Knowles' principles of adult learning state adult learners tend to be:
    a. Unmotivated.
    b. Lacking in self-direction
    c. Practical and goal-oriented
    d. Insecure

10. Identify the smoking cessation medication you must monitor carefully because of its dangerous side- effects:
    a. Nicotine nasal spray
    b. Bupropion (Zyban®)
    c. Nicotine inhaler
    d. Varenicline (Chantix®)

11. The patient payer is a client who legally agrees to pay the Nurse Practitioner directly for providing a specific service, which is a:
    a. Fee-for-service system
    b. Third-party system
    c. Contracted service system
    d. Second-party system

12. Identify the behavioral change model that predicts a person takes a health action to avoid negative consequences, believing the action will prevent a negative outcome:
    a. Theory of reasoned action
    b. Theory of planned behavior
    c. Stress appraisal and coping theory
    d. Health belief model

13. Identify the members of the healthcare institution who are responsible for identifying performance improvement projects:
    a. Administrative staff
    b. Nursing team leaders
    c. All staff
    d. Physicians

14. Your patient is a 66-year-old male receiving Medicare. He is discharged with an open, draining chest wound that he cannot care for independently because of poor vision. His 14-year-old grandson lives with him. The best solution is:
    a. Transfer your patient to an extended care facility
    b. Keep your patient hospitalized until his wound heals
    c. Teach your patient's 14-year-old grandson to provide wound care
    d. Refer him to a health agency that provides in-home care

15. Your patient is a 65-year-old male. You assess his jugular venous pressure by elevating his head to 45⬚ and turning it to the right. The height of the jugular vein pulsation is 5 cm above his sternal angle, which may indicate:
    a. Increased pressure in his right atrium and right heart failure
    b. Increased pressure in his left atrium and left heart failure
    c. Mitral stenosis
    d. A normal reading

16. Your patient receives unfractionated heparin therapy. His baseline platelet count was 120,000 mm^3. After 5 days of treatment, his platelet count suddenly drops to 45,000 mm^3, suggesting heparin-induced thrombocytopenia. Your patient is at risk for:
    a. Hemorrhage
    b. Thrombosis and vessel occlusion
    c. Shock
    d. Infection

17. A patient with an internal locus of control probably believes:
    a. His family will take care of him
    b. His health is a matter of fate
    c. He is in control of his health
    d. The doctor and nurses control the outcome of his disease

18. Your infant patient had surgical closure of his ductus arteriosus. Blood pressure in his head and upper extremities increases. Blood pressure to his lower extremities decreases. These symptoms may indicate:
    a. Tetralogy of Fallot
    b. Pulmonic stenosis
    c. Coarctation of the aorta
    d. Ventricular septal defect

19. Your patient spends half the year in one state and half in another state. He wants to complete an advance directive. Select the best approach:
    a. Check the laws for both states; complete two separate advance directives, each complying with one state's regulations
    b. Complete only one advance directive, as all states have the same regulations
    c. Tell family members his wishes, so an advance directive is unnecessary
    d. Store the original advance directive(s) in a safety deposit box

20. The goal of an exercise stress test is to:
    a. Raise the heart rate to 200% of predicted for age and gender
    b. Raise the heart to 50% of predicted for age and gender
    c. Raise the heart rate between 80% and 90% of predicted for age and gender
    d. Raise the heart rate above 100% of predicted for age and gender

21. Select the most effective, efficient teaching method for teaching a group of patients about lifestyle modifications related to hypertension:
    a. Computer-assisted instruction
    b. Group lecture only
    c. Group lecture and discussion
    d. One-on-one instruction

22. Identify the coding system the Centers for Medicare and Medicaid (CMS) requires you to use to obtain reimbursement for nursing services from Medicare:
    a. Current Procedural Terminology (CPT)
    b. Healthcare Common Procedure Coding System (HCPCS)
    c. International Statistical Classification of Diseases and Related Health Problems (ICD)
    d. Diagnosis-Related Groups (DRG)

23. Your patient receives digoxin and furosemide daily. The doctor prescribes tetracycline for your patient's rosacea. Subsequently, your patient develops nausea, vomiting, and tachycardia. Identify the MOST likely cause:
    a. Digitalis toxicity
    b. Allergic response to tetracycline
    c. Drug interaction between furosemide and tetracycline
    d. Superinfection

24. The normal volume of air inhaled and exhaled during each breath while at rest is the:
    a. Inspiratory reserve volume
    b. Expiratory reserve volume
    c. Residual volume
    d. Tidal volume

25. Choose the most appropriate educational tool for your English-speaking patient, who is illiterate:
    a. A children's book
    b. Handouts prepared at the third grade level
    c. Computerized instruction
    d. A video

26. Your nursing team leader delegates tasks to unlicensed assistive personnel. Identify the person(s) responsible for patient outcomes:
    a. The unlicensed delegates who complete the tasks
    b. Both the team leader and the unlicensed personnel who complete the tasks
    c. The team leader who delegates the tasks
    d. The administrative staff

27. Your patient is a 65-year-old female. She is 5 feet 4 inches tall and weighs 180 lb. She has mild congestive heart failure and diabetes type 2. She followed an 800-calorie/day diet for two weeks and performed 5 to 8 minutes of daily exercise. She lost 15 pounds. Choose the best advice for your patient:
    a. Increase your caloric intake, exercise, and maintain your weight loss at 1 to 2 pounds per week
    b. Maintain this effective diet and exercise plan
    c. Increase your caloric intake to maintain your weight loss at 5 pounds per week
    d. Maintain this same diet plan, but increase your exercise

28. Your patient is a 40-year-old male with a possible myocardial infarction. He sweats profusely during his electrocardiogram. Identify the artifact, if any, that results from diaphoresis:
    a. Baseline drift
    b. 60 Hz
    c. Movement
    d. None

29. Name the support system that includes organizations and agencies providing goods and services:
    a. Formal
    b. Semiformal
    c. Informal
    d. Family

30. Identify the MOST important component when you develop evidence-based guidelines:
    a. An evidence review
    b. The opinion of your Chief of Staff
    c. A staff survey
    d. The cost-effectiveness of your guidelines

31. Identify the law that provides improved access to transportation for older adults and Native Americans:
    a. Emergency Medical Treatment and Active Labor Act (EMTALA)
    b. Omnibus Budget Reconciliation Act (OBRA)
    c. Americans with Disabilities Act (ADA)
    d. Older Americans Act (OAA)

32. Identify the right included in the *Patients' Bill of Rights*:
    a. The right to affordable healthcare
    b. The right to pain control
    c. The right to sue
    d. The right of access to the latest medical technology

33. Your patient is a 22-year-old male, diagnosed with Buerger disease. His primary non-pharmacological treatment should be to:
    a. Avoid alcohol
    b. Stop smoking
    c. Increase exercise
    d. Lose weight

34. Your patient is 13 years old. Before receiving chemotherapy for her leukemia, she states, "There is no point in having this treatment." Choose the best nursing response:
    a. "You must have chemotherapy in order to get well."
    b. "Do you believe the treatment isn't helping you?"
    c. "You should talk to your doctor about that."
    d. "Your parents have decided you should have chemotherapy."

35. Your patient is a female infant, diagnosed with Tay Sachs (TS) disease. To inherit TS, the child must have received an abnormal gene on chromosome 15 from each of her parents. This form of inheritance is:
    a. Autosomal recessive
    b. Autosomal dominant
    c. X-linked recessive
    d. Y-linked

36. Your patient has chronic knee pain from osteoarthritis. She wants to try complementary therapy to reduce her use of analgesics. Identify the complementary therapy MOST likely to reduce her pain:
    a. Orthomolecular therapy
    b. Homeopathy
    c. Aromatherapy
    d. Acupuncture

37. Bowen's family system theory states:
    a. A change in one person's behavior affects the others in the family
    b. The basic family unit is two people; adding a third is disruptive and results in conflict
    c. People in the same family have similar needs for external approval
    d. Family members function independently

38. If a mother has an X-linked dominant disease, she can transmit the disease to:
    a. Her daughters only
    b. Her sons only
    c. Half of her sons and half of her daughters
    d. None of her offspring

39. A newly-hired nurse assists her team leader with an IV insertion. The team leader drops the sterile catheter onto the bed linens, picks up the contaminated catheter, and prepares for insertion. Choose the new hire's best response:
    a. Wait until the team leader finishes the procedure, then ask why she used the contaminated catheter
    b. Report the team leader's behavior to the nursing supervisor after the catheter is inserted
    c. Say nothing to anyone, as the linens were clean
    d. Immediately say, "The catheter was contaminated when it fell. Would you like me to get another setup or stay with the patient while you get it?"

40. Your patient is a 12-year-old girl. The doctor sutured a 2 cm cut on her forehead. You tell her mother to bring her back, so you can remove her sutures in:
    a. Two days
    b. Five days
    c. 10 days
    d. 14 days

41. The Health Insurance Portability and Accountability Act:
    a. Addresses the rights of the individual, as they relate to privacy of health information
    b. Requires national standards for electronic health records
    c. Provides the right to continued health insurance coverage for those who lose or change employment
    d. All of the above

42. The best determinant of the effectiveness of patient education is:
    a. Patient satisfaction
    b. The patient's ability to correctly demonstrate the procedure
    c. The patient's ability to explain the procedure and demonstrate understanding
    d. The patient's behavior modification and compliance rates

43. A bat bit your 18-year-old female patient's hand, leaving a small puncture wound. She dropped the bat while trying to remove it from her apartment. The bat escaped, so it cannot be tested. Identify the MOST important treatment:
    a. Antibiotics
    b. Analgesia
    c. Wound irrigation
    d. Rabies post-exposure prophylaxis (PEP)

44. Your 26-year-old female patient states her mother, maternal grandmother, and sister all had breast cancer. Choose the MOST important initial test for her:
    a. Mammogram
    b. Ultrasound
    c. Genetic predictive testing
    d. Chest x-ray

45. Choose the patient who is NOT a member of a vulnerable population, in relation to research studies:
    a. A woman with advanced ovarian cancer
    b. A person incarcerated in prison
    c. An adult with cognitive impairment
    d. A 7-year-old child

46. Your patient is a 15-year old girl dying of cancer. Her mother claims the doctor misdiagnosed her daughter's condition and she demands a different doctor. Identify the stage of grief the mother is in, according to Kübler-Ross:
    a. Denial
    b. Anger
    c. Bargaining
    d. Depression

47. Your patient is a 16-year-old boy, who sprained his ankle playing basketball. Select the treatment MOST appropriate for his grade II inversion injury:
    a. Analgesia only
    b. Cast application
    c. Surgical repair
    d. RICE (rest, ice, compress, elevate)

48. Your patient is a 50-year-old male with hyperlipidemia. His lipid profile is LDL 135 mg/dL, HDL 55 mg/dL, and triglycerides 200 mg/dL. Identify the lipid result that is MOST abnormal, if any:
    a. LDL
    b. HDL
    c. Triglycerides
    d. All results are within normal range

49. Your patient is a 36-year-old female marathon runner. She developed increasing pain during training and point tenderness to percussion of her shin. Her x-ray is negative for fracture. Indicate the next logical test, if any:
    a. None
    b. MRI
    c. Muscle biopsy
    d. Bone scan

50. Select the best strategy to help your patient overcome her feelings of low self-esteem, related to chronic illness and loss of autonomy:
    a. Praise the patient constantly for any activities
    b. Tell the patient she has no reason to feel so depressed
    c. Provide opportunities for your patient to make decisions
    d. Avoid talking to your patient about her feelings

51. Identify the organization responsible for outlining the Nurse Practitioner's scope of practice:
    a. The American Nurses Association
    b. The American Nurses Credentialing Center (ANCC)
    c. The individual state's Board of Nursing and Nurse Practice Act
    d. The American Academy of Nurse Practitioners

52. Identify the Medicare-approved program(s) that pays a set amount for patient care, depending on the diagnosis-related group (DRG):
    a. Preferred provider organization (PPO)
    b. Prospective payment system (PPS)
    c. Private service pay-for-service Medicare plans
    d. Specialty plans

53. Your patient is a 50-year-old, overweight male with a third degree burn on his left arm. He had wound debridement and a skin graft. Select the dietary modification MOST important to promote his healing:
    a. Decreased fats
    b. Increased protein
    c. Increased carbohydrate
    d. Decreased calories

54. Select the strategy most likely to help your patient come to terms with the change in his self-image resulting from his large surgical scar:
    a. Provide acceptance, and show no revulsion or negative feelings about your patient's appearance
    b. Provide personal care, rather than having the patient engage in self-care
    c. Discourage your patient from looking at his altered body part
    d. Tell your patient how lucky he is, and reassure him that he is recovering

55. Your patient is a 10-year-old African American boy. He is obese, with slightly elevated blood pressure. He develops enuresis. Select the MOST important initial screening test(s) for him:
    a. Blood glucose and Hemoglobin A1c
    b. Renal function tests
    c. Thyroid function test
    d. Electrocardiogram

56. Your patient is an 82-year-old female recovering from a hip fracture. She is ready for discharge from an acute care hospital, but needs physiotherapy. She lives alone and has no visiting caregiver. She has numerous comorbidities. The MOST appropriate referral for her is a:
    a. Hospice
    b. Home health agency
    c. Skilled nursing facility
    d. Residential care facility

57. Screening for cervical cancer by Papanicolaou (Pap) smear is indicated for:
    a. All females over age 16 or within 5 years of becoming sexually active
    b. All females over age 18 or within 5 years of becoming sexually active
    c. Only females who state they are currently sexually active
    d. All females over age 21 or within 3 years of becoming sexually active

58. The American Medical Association states the doctor must communicate all of the following to the patient when obtaining informed consent, EXCEPT the:
    a. Risks and benefits of NOT having a treatment or procedure
    b. Explanation of the diagnosis
    c. Nature and reason for the treatment or procedure
    d. Cost comparisons

59. You are interviewing a 40-year-old Chinese woman. She seems relaxed and answers all your questions fully. However, she keeps her eyes downcast and does not make eye contact. Her body language probably indicates:
    a. Respect
    b. Fear
    c. Depression
    d. Dishonesty

60. Your female patient has a single wart on her arm. Select the MOST appropriate initial treatment:
    a. Cryotherapy
    b. Excision
    c. CO2 laser ablation
    d. Pulse dye laser ablation

61. Identify the program that provides people with low income with payment assistance for medical care:
    a. Medicaid
    b. Medicare
    c. Social Security (SS)
    d. Supplemental Security Income (SSI)

62. You are teaching your patient to manage his tracheostomy care, using written directions and a video. Your patient ignores the teaching aids, but picks up the equipment, looks at each part, and tries to figure it out independently. Your patient's learning style is probably:
    a. Auditory
    b. Visual
    c. Kinesthetic
    d. Mixed

63. You are researching the most effective method of reducing urinary tract infections in hospitalized patients. Your first step is to:
    a. Develop a list of possible interventions
    b. Interview staff members
    c. Develop a list of possible causes
    d. Complete a literature review

64. Your patient is a 20-year-old woman, on life support following a traffic accident. Her parents divorced when she was 12. Her father had legal custody. She lived with him until two months ago, then moved in with her fiancé. Her mother has a signed, *Durable Power of Attorney for Health Care*, allowing her to make decisions on her unconscious daughter's behalf. However, for the past year mother and daughter were estranged. Identify the legal decision-maker for continuing or stopping life support:

    a. Her fiancé makes the decision, because they lived together
    b. Her mother makes the decision, based on the Durable Power of Attorney
    c. Her father makes the decision, because he had legal custody
    d. The Bioethics Committee asks the court to decide

65. Your patient is a 15-year-old boy. He is tall, thin, with abnormally long arms and legs, pectus carinatum (pigeon chest), mild scoliosis, flat feet, a long face, a highly arched palate, and crowded teeth. He wants your clearance to play football. You screen the child for:

    a. Aortic stenosis
    b. Aortic dilatation
    c. Mitral valve stenosis
    d. Rheumatic fever

66. Name the regular assessment you perform for your patients receiving phenytoin (Dilantin®):

    a. Psychiatric
    b. Gynecological/Genitourinary
    c. Dental
    d. Dermatological

67. A learner outcome for teaching patients with hyperlipidemia about diet is:

    a. Your patient can explain the difference between LDL and HDL
    b. Your patient can list foods containing saturated and unsaturated fats
    c. Your patient plans to stop using olive oil for cooking
    d. Your patient states his goal is to increase his triglyceride level above 200 mg/dL

68. Your patient is a 32-year-old female with hypotension. She complains of chronic weakness, fatigue, nausea, and licorice craving. The skin of her axillae, inferior breast surfaces, and buccal mucosa are hyperpigmented. The most likely diagnosis is:

    a. Addison disease
    b. Cushing syndrome
    c. Hypothyroidism
    d. Hyperthyroidism

69. Your patient is a 70-year-old widower, hospitalized for malnutrition. He has poor vision and rheumatoid arthritis. He lives alone in a large home. Since his wife died, he eats primarily snack foods because they are easy to access. His condition is now stable. Select the MOST appropriate referral on discharge:

    a. A skilled nursing facility (SNF)
    b. Meals-on-Wheels
    c. Medicaid
    d. Adult Protective Services

70. The best method to evaluate your patient's educational outcomes after teaching him a procedure is to:
    a. Ask your patient to demonstrate for you
    b. Ask your patient for feedback
    c. Give your patient an oral test
    d. Give your patient a written test

71. Your patient is a child with rubeola (measles), hospitalized when it is complicated by encephalitis. Identify the precautions required for measles, according to the CDC's *2007 Guideline for Isolation Precautions*:
    a. Standard precautions
    b. Airborne precautions
    c. Droplet precautions
    d. Contact precautions

72. Name the federal law allowing parents to provide insurance coverage for their children on a family policy until age 26:
    a. Americans with Disabilities Act (ADA)
    b. Older Americans Act (OAA)
    c. Affordable Care Act
    d. Omnibus Budget Reconciliation Act (OBRA)

73. Identify the immunization vaccine recommended for patients 60 and older:
    a. Pneumococcal polysaccharide-23
    b. Hepatitis A
    c. Hepatitis B
    d. Herpes zoster

74. Your patient is a 45-year-old bipolar female, on lithium maintenance. She reports chronic fatigue, irregular periods, hoarseness, low body temperature (96.8⬜ F), weight gain, thickened skin, and hair loss. Identify her MOST important initial laboratory test(s):
    a. Estrogen level
    b. Complete blood count and blood culture
    c. Thyroid function tests
    d. Liver function test

75. You enter your patient's room after he spoke with his doctor. You find your patient shaking and distraught. Select the best nursing response:
    a. "What's wrong?"
    b. "Do you want me to call your family?"
    c. "You are shaking and seem worried."
    d. "You don't need to worry. Everything will be all right."

76. Identify the vaccination advised for girls between ages 11 and 12:
    a. Human papillomavirus vaccine (Gardasil®)
    b. Rotavirus
    c. Hepatitis A
    d. Measles, mumps, and rubella (MMR)

77. The CDC's *2007 Guideline for Isolation Precautions* calls a wound infection developed by the patient at home, while receiving care from a home health agency, a:
    a. Nosocomial infection
    b. Healthcare-associated infection
    c. Non-healthcare-associated infection
    d. Community-associated infection

78. Your patient has gastroenteritis and severe dehydration, with more than 15% fluid loss. His symptoms will include:
    a. Dry mouth and increased thirst
    b. Dizziness, lethargy, reduced skin turgor, and orthostatic hypotension
    c. Resting hypotension, confusion, tachycardia, and oliguria
    d. Marked hypotension and anuria, in addition to other symptoms

79. Identify the patient response during an interview that allows you to elicit the most important information:
    a. Verbal responses
    b. Non-verbal responses
    c. Silence
    d. Both verbal and non-verbal responses

80. Select the term that describes the biological effects of drugs over time:
    a. Pharmacokinetics
    b. Pharmacodynamics
    c. Half-time
    d. Effect-site equilibrium

81. Interactive software applications that provide information to physicians or other healthcare providers to help with healthcare decisions are called:
    a. Computerized physician/provider order entry (CPOE)
    b. Computerized notification systems
    c. Electronic medical record (EMR)
    d. Clinical decision support systems (CDSS)

82. The test that helps to differentiate between diastolic and systolic heart failure by determining ejection fraction is the:
    a. Chest x-ray
    b. Echocardiogram
    c. Angiograms
    d. Electrocardiogram

83. You are on the unit, completing an Admission History for your Hispanic patient. He speaks very little English. Your best recourse is to:
    a. Ask the patient's 12-year-old son, who is fluent in English, to translate for you
    b. Use sign language and pictures to supplement your questions
    c. Arrange for a professional translator to attend the intake
    d. Ask the patient's wife, who speaks fair English, to answer your questions on her husband's behalf

84. The CDC recommends contact precautions in addition to standard precautions for patients infected with:
    a. Hepatitis B
    b. *Mycobacterium tuberculosis*
    c. *Haemophilus influenzae*
    d. *Clostridium difficile*

85. Your patient is a 16-year-old girl, hospitalized with severe depression. She has urinary incontinence, although her urinary system is normal. The MOST appropriate nursing diagnosis is:
    a. Functional urinary incontinence
    b. Stress urinary incontinence
    c. Overflow urinary incontinence
    d. Urge urinary incontinence

86. Choose the diet necessary to treat celiac disease:
    a. Low fat
    b. Lactose (dairy) free
    c. Gluten free
    d. Low carbohydrate

87. Fill-in-the-blank. According to Piaget's theory of cognitive development, children engage in magical thinking and show egocentrism during the _____ stage:
    a. Sensorimotor
    b. Preoperational
    c. Concrete operational
    d. Formal operational

88. Name the dementia assessment tool that requires the patient to remember and repeat the names of three common objects, and to draw the face of a clock with all 12 numbers, with its hands indicating the time specified by the examiner:
    a. Mini-mental state exam (MMSE)
    b. Mini-cog
    c. Digit Repetition Test
    d. Confusion Assessment Method

89. The first-line diuretic for treatment of mild hypertension is a:
    a. Loop diuretic
    b. Potassium-sparing diuretic
    c. Thiazide diuretic
    d. Combined loop diuretic and potassium-sparing diuretic

90. You must safely inject three different but compatible drugs into your patient's IV tube. Each drug is supplied in its own single-dose vial. The CDC requires you to:
    a. Use the same needle and syringe for all three drugs
    b. Use the same needle but clean syringes for the three drugs
    c. Use clean needles but the same syringe for the three drugs
    d. Use a clean needle and clean syringe for each of the three drugs

91. Name the theory that proposes children learn by interacting with adults and their peers, and through modeling behavior, but are capable of making behavioral choices:
     a. Kohlberg's theory of moral development
     b. Bandura's theory of social learning
     c. Watson's theory of behaviorism
     d. Chess and Thomas's temperament theory

92. Your patient complains of pain. You administer morphine, as per the doctor's PRN order. You must document administration of morphine:
     a. Immediately
     b. Within 1 to 2 hours
     c. Within 4 hours
     d. By the end of your shift

93. Your patient is a 13-year-old girl with a viral upper respiratory infection. Initially, she had a dry, hacking cough that worsened at night. It became productive after two days. Her cough has persisted for 12 days, but she remains afebrile. Select the MOST appropriate initial action:
     a. Order sputum culture and sensitivities
     b. Ask your patient to return in one week for follow-up
     c. Prescribe a course of antibiotics
     d. Prescribe an antiviral medication

94. Your renal patient has ventricular arrhythmia, increasing EKG changes, weakness, ascending paralysis, hyperreflexia, diarrhea, and increasing confusion. The MOST likely cause is:
     a. Hyperkalemia
     b. Hypokalemia
     c. Hypocalcemia
     d. Hypercalcemia

95. Your patient is a mentally-alert 80-year-old woman, hospitalized for an extended period. Her husband is visiting her and the door is ajar. A visitor complains to you that she saw the husband fondling his wife, as she walked by your patient's room. Select your MOST appropriate action:
     a. Explain to your patient and her husband that their behavior is inappropriate
     b. Call the husband from the room and explain that his behavior is inappropriate
     c. Close your patient's door to allow them privacy
     d. Ask the husband to leave

96. Your patient is a 56-year-old female, who is frequently constipated. Increasing fiber and fluids in her diet did not alleviate her constipation. She takes occasional laxatives and water enemas to prevent impaction. Her colonoscopy is normal. Select the next treatment that is MOST appropriate:
     a. A daily stool softener, such as Colace®
     b. A daily bulk former, such as Metamucil®
     c. A small, daily dose of laxative, such as Milk of Magnesia®
     d. Routine saline enemas

97. The timed-up-and-go (TUG) test assesses:
   a. Muscle strength
   b. Cognitive status
   c. Mobility and risk of falls
   d. Walking speed

98. Your patient is a 30-year-old, malnourished male, with slight fever and tachycardia. He complains of frequent nosebleeds, abdominal pain, and nausea. You observe miosis, finger burns, repeated sniffing, and a slight cough. He has no needle marks. Identify the MOST likely substance he is abusing:
   a. Cocaine
   b. Heroin
   c. Marijuana
   d. Methadone

99. Your patient is a 10-year-old boy, whose parents are Jehovah Witnesses. He has life-threatening hypovolemic shock, requiring blood transfusions. On admission, his parents indicated, "No transfusions." Choose your most appropriate FIRST action:
   a. Contact Risk Management to ask for advice
   b. Tell the parents their child will die if they refuse blood transfusions
   c. Contact Child Protective Services to request intervention
   d. Provide full information to the parents, and allow them to express their feelings

100. Your patient is a 32-year-old, bipolar female on lithium. She appears weak and tremulous. She complains of "severe flu." Her lithium level is 2 mEq/L. Select your MOST appropriate action:
   a. Discontinue lithium until her blood level is less than 1.5 mEq/L
   b. Maintain her current lithium dosage; prescribe rest and fluids
   c. Increase lithium, and monitor her blood level until it exceeds 2.5 mEq/L
   d. Maintain her current lithium dosage and order a complete blood count

101. Nursing informatics is:
   a. The general study of information
   b. The integration of nursing, computer, and information sciences in the management of data and information.
   c. Statistical analyses of nursing effectiveness
   d. Computerized record keeping

102. Identify the chemical that causes serotonin syndrome (rapid alterations in BP, diaphoresis, nausea, vomiting, muscle rigidity, seizures, and coma) when combined with a selective serotonin reuptake inhibitor (SSRI):
   a. NSAIDs
   b. Monoamine oxidase inhibitors
   c. Digoxin
   d. Alcohol

103. Your patient is a 15-year-old, sexually active girl. She uses the rhythm method to prevent pregnancy. You should:
    a. Advise her to stop having sex because she is a minor
    b. Tell her parents their daughter is sexually active
    c. Educate her about birth control methods
    d. Refer her to a counselor

104. You live in the same apartment building as your female patient. She is very ill, so asks if you would mind bringing her a few personal items and her mail. You should:
    a. Agree to pick up the items, since you are neighbors
    b. Refuse, saying it is against hospital policy
    c. Ask the apartment manager to gather her items and mail and deliver them
    d. State you cannot do so personally, but will help her to call a friend or family member

105. Your patient is a 70-year-old male with peripheral venous insufficiency. His symptoms probably include:
    a. Aching, cramping leg pain; brownish discoloration of his ankles and shin (anterior tibia)
    b. Intermediate to severe constant leg pain, with rubor on dependency
    c. Deep circular, necrotic ulcers on his toe tips, toe webs, heels, or other pressure areas
    d. Weak or absent pedal pulses and minimal edema

106. Your patient is a breastfeeding mother. She complains of pain when her infant latches onto her nipple. You should:
    a. Advise her to rub her nipples with a rough cloth to "toughen" them
    b. Observe her breastfeeding and educate her about correct infant positioning and latching on
    c. Advise her that pain is normal and usually passes with time
    d. Advise her to use a nipple shield to prevent pain

107. Your patient is a 30-year-old female. She was beaten and raped six months ago, while leaving work. She returned to work soon after the attack, but now refuses to go to work. She appears fearful but refuses to talk about the rape. She avoids friends and has little interest in formerly enjoyed activities. She sleeps poorly and sometimes awakes screaming. She has outburst of temper, startles easily, and appears to "space-out" at times. Her MOST likely diagnosis is:
    a. Schizophrenia
    b. Post-traumatic stress disorder
    c. Chronic depression
    d. Bi-polar disorder

108. Your patient has cancer. He is very decisive and opinionated about his chemotherapy treatment. He wants to know the results of every test. When his white count falls, he becomes upset and begins makes demands about his diet and care. His communication style is classified as:
    a. Expressor
    b. Driver
    c. Relater
    d. Analytical

109. Your female patient breastfeeds her infant. She develops a blocked milk duct, featuring a painful, localized lump. Choose her MOST appropriate initial treatment:
    a. Antibiotic therapy
    b. Avoid breastfeeding on her affected side
    c. Hand express her milk, and massage the breast lump under a warm shower
    d. Apply ice packs to her inflamed breast

110. Erikson's theory of psychosocial development states the conflict typical of young adults older than 18 is:
    a. Intimacy vs. isolation
    b. Autonomy vs. shame and doubt
    c. Generativity vs. stagnation
    d. Trust vs. mistrust

111. You documented administration of Lasix 40 mg in the wrong patient's chart. The proper procedure for correcting your charting error is to:
    a. Cover the charting error with Wite-out® corrector fluid
    b. Draw several lines through the charting error
    c. Draw one ink line through the charting error, write "Error" above it, and initial and date your change
    d. Leave the incorrect entry intact but write an explanation beneath it

112. Your patient has Broca's (non-fluent) aphasia, caused by damage to the frontal lobe of his brain. Choose the MOST effective communication approach for this patient:
    a. Use pictures, diagrams, charts, and gestures
    b. Speak slowly and clearly, and let the patient use a picture chart to respond
    c. Gesture and provide the patient with writing materials or a letter board to respond
    d. Gesture only

113. Your patient is a 36-year-old male, who fell on his elbow. It is extremely painful and flexed at a 60⯑ angle. He suffers arm muscle spasms, but his circulation is good. Your initial treatment should be:
    a. Gently straighten his arm to 90⯑ flexion, and secure it with a splint
    b. Splint his arm securely, without attempting to change the degree of flexion
    c. Gently put his elbow through range of motion exercises to determine the extent of his injury
    d. Apply a compression dressing from his fingers to above his elbow

114. Your patient is a 60-year-old male construction worker. He remodeled old homes and businesses for 40 years. Recently, he lost weight and developed a cough, dyspnea, and hoarseness. His right chest wall is chronically painful, and is exacerbated by coughing. He never smoked. His MOST likely diagnosis is:
    a. Asthma
    b. Lung cancer (small cell or non-small cell)
    c. Chronic obstructive pulmonary disease (COPD)
    d. Mesothelioma

115. Identify the drug that promotes weight loss by preventing fat absorption:
   a. Benzphetamine (Didrex®)
   b. Diethylpropion (Tenuate®)
   c. Orlistat (Xenical®, Alli®)
   d. Phentermine (Adipex-P®, Kraftobese®)

116. Your patient is a 17-year-old girl. She confides that she is depressed and has suicidal ideation. She asks you not to tell her parents. Select the action MOST appropriate for this confidentiality dilemma:
   a. Respect the girl's right to confidentiality; do not tell her parents
   b. Call her parents after the visit to tell them about their daughter's depression
   c. Tell her parents the girl needs counseling to deal with "peer pressure"
   d. Insist on telling her parents with the girl present; support the girl and help the family to discuss the issue

117. Your patient is a 22-year-old gay male, who is a victim of domestic violence by his partner. Your MOST appropriate initial response is:
   a. "You should notify the police."
   b. "Domestic violence relates to violence against females."
   c. "Are you in immediate danger, and is your abuser on the premises?"
   d. "What type of abuse are you talking about?"

118. Your patient is a 48-year-old female with normal menses. She takes birth control pills, and H_2-histamine receptor blockers to decrease her gastric hydrochloric acid. She develops anemia, a sore tongue, anorexia, nausea, vomiting, paresthesias with reduced sense of position and vibration, ataxia, muscle weakness, and mild confusion. Her MOST likely diagnosis is:
   a. Iron deficiency anemia
   b. Pernicious anemia (Vitamin B12/cobalamin deficiency)
   c. Folic acid deficiency
   d. Aplastic anemia

119. The optimal irrigation pressure for an open, contaminated wound is:
   a. Less than 4 psi
   b. 4 to 9 psi
   c. 10 to 15 psi
   d. Greater than 15 psi

120. Your elderly female patient fractured her hip because she became dizzy and fell. She stopped taking her antihypertensives because she cannot afford them. She supports her son and his family, who moved in with her six months ago. Her son now manages her financial affairs. Her case is an example of:
   a. Neglect
   b. Physical abuse
   c. Psychological abuse
   d. Financial abuse

121. Identify your MOST important consideration when deciding where to place computer terminals, as your office converts to computerized record keeping:
a. Terminals should be easily accessible
b. Terminals must be placed where others cannot read notes as they are typed
c. Terminals should be placed by patients' bedsides
d. Terminals should be positioned so the nurse can enter information while standing

122. Select the MOST effective dressing type for a full-thickness wound with undermining, tunneling, and excessive drainage:
a. Alginate
b. Hydrogel
c. Hydrocolloid
d. Semi-permeable film

123. Your patient is a 4-year-old boy, hospitalized for inguinal herniorrhaphy. Select the MOST appropriate teaching method to prepare this child:
a. Puppet, doll, and needle play
b. Video demonstration
c. Picture book explanation
d. Verbal explanation

124. Identify the MOST accurate laboratory test to evaluate *acute* changes in nutritional status:
a. Total protein
b. Albumin
c. Prealbumin
d. Transferrin

125. Anticipatory guidance during early adolescence (ages 11 to 14) should include discussion of:
a. Methods to avoid gangs, tobacco, drugs, alcohol, and abusive relationships
b. Sexual responsibility: Abstinence, birth control
c. Relationships and risk-taking behavior
d. Future goals

126. Identify the patient most at risk for developing a weight-related disorder, such as hypertension or diabetes:
a. Female with a waist circumference of 37 inches
b. Male with waist circumference of 39 inches
c. Male with a BMI of 20
d. Female with a BMI of 24.5

127. Your patient is a 48-year-old, overweight male, who lives alone. He complains of chronic sleepiness, despite sleeping 8 to 10 hours nightly. His other symptoms include mild depression and markedly decreased libido. He has 3 to 4 alcoholic drinks each evening. He states his snoring sometimes "jerks" him awake. Choose the initial diagnostic test MOST indicated by his profile:
    a. Androgen level
    b. Nocturnal polysomnography
    c. Liver function tests
    d. Proctoscopy

128. The current screening guidelines for colorectal cancer in the 50 to 75 age group require:
    a. High-sensitivity fecal occult blood test (FOBT) annually and colonoscopy every 5 years
    b. High-sensitivity fecal occult blood test (FOBT) bi-annually and colonoscopy every 5 years
    c. Flexible sigmoidoscopy every 5 years and colonoscopy every 10 years
    d. High-sensitivity FOBT annually, flexible sigmoidoscopy every 5 years, and colonoscopy every 10 years

129. A homeless, unemployed woman brings her three-year-old daughter to the hospital because she is very concerned. The child had a cough and fever for two weeks, which her mother treated with acetaminophen and cough syrup provided by a friend. The child's diagnosis is pneumonia. Choose the primary factor MOST likely to have caused the mother to delay bringing her child for care:
    a. Poverty
    b. Lack of transportation
    c. Lack of healthcare availability
    d. Neglect

130. Your patient is a 65-year-old female with diabetes type 2. She is scheduled for magnetic resonance imaging (MRI) with gadolinium contrast. Name the laboratory blood test indicated prior to her MRI:
    a. Serum glucose
    b. Creatinine clearance
    c. Thyroid function
    d. Serum electrolytes

131. A caregiver providing long-term care for a hospice patient with a terminal or chronic illness, such as Alzheimer disease, may be eligible for:
    a. Twenty-four hour/day nursing assistance for 10 days
    b. Payment for hours spent caring for the patient
    c. Respite care
    d. A housekeeper

132. Your patient is a 26-year-old, sexually active female. She wants a prescription for isotretinoin (Accutane®) to cure her severe acne. She had a negative pregnancy test two weeks ago. For three months, she took progesterone-only birth control pills and used a diaphragm with lubricant as a back-up method. Identify the changes in birth control methods, if any, necessary under the IPLEDGE protocol for isotretinoin:
  a. The two forms of birth control are acceptable
  b. She must change to a birth control pill containing estrogen
  c. She must change to a birth control pill containing estrogen and use spermicide with her diaphragm
  d. She may stay on the progesterone-only birth control pill, but must use spermicide with her diaphragm

133. Identify the indicator that does NOT require the nurse to perform directly-observed therapy (DOT) for treatment of tuberculosis:
  a. Non-English speaking patient
  b. Co-morbidity with HIV with concurrent treatment
  c. Cognitive impairment
  d. Homelessness

134. Your patient is a 38-year-old, overweight woman. She complains of recurrent episodes of severe right upper quadrant or epigastric pain, persisting two to six hours per episode, sometimes associated with nausea. Choose the initial test MOST indicated to confirm a diagnosis of cholecystitis:
  a. Abdominal MRI
  b. Liver function tests
  c. Cholangiogram
  d. Abdominal ultrasound

135. Your patient is a 16-year-old football player, who was practicing in 90ºF weather. His signs and symptoms of heat exhaustion include diaphoresis, nausea, dizziness, and muscle cramps. His heart rate is 100 bpm. His temperature 99.6ºF. He is weak but alert. Along with rehydration, choose the MOST appropriate cooling method:
  a. Alcohol bath
  b. Ice bath immersion for 5 to 10 minutes
  c. Intravascular cooling with cold IV fluids
  d. Cold packs on his neck, groin, and axillae

136. You generated a problem list for your 59-year-old patient and are developing goals. One problem is cardiac arrhythmia with tachycardia, and the goal is "Pulse rate will not exceed 90 at rest." The aim of this goal is:
  a. Maintaining status quo
  b. Providing palliation
  c. Preventing deterioration
  d. Providing resolution

137. An example of tertiary prevention is:
  a. Getting an annual flu immunization
  b. Taking daily low-dose Aspirin after a heart attack
  c. Having routine mammograms
  d. Attending Alcoholics Anonymous

138. Your patient is a 78-year-old male with a history of diverticulosis. He develops steady pain in his left lower quadrant, constipation, tenesmus, fever, and abdominal distention. Choose the initial test necessary to confirm a diagnosis of diverticulitis:
    a. Stool for occult blood
    b. Abdominal CT
    c. Barium enema
    d. White blood cell count

139. Identify the CORRECT statement regarding transient tic disorder:
    a. Tics must be present for four weeks but no longer than one year
    b. Vocal tics are more common than movement tics
    c. Tic behavior is more common in the spring and summer
    d. Tics continue during all stages of sleep

140. A Medicare patient may receive hospice care if:
    a. The patient requests Hospice care
    b. The patient is eligible for Medicare B and has a terminal illness
    c. The patient is eligible for Medicare B and a physician certifies the patient has a life expectancy of one year or less
    d. The patient is eligible for Medicare A, and a physician certifies the patient has a life expectancy of six months or less

141. You are assessing a 14-month-old child for developmentally appropriate communication. The child should be able to:
    a. Say a few words, such as "Mama" and "Dada" and imitate some animal sounds
    b. Use an expressive vocabulary of four to six words, but understand many more words, and point to something desired, such as a toy
    c. Use an expressive vocabulary of seven to 20 words, and point to five body parts
    d. Combine two words to create simple sentences or phrases

142. Identify the communication model that focuses on observation, feelings, needs, and requests (OFNR):
    a. Rosenberg's non-violent communication
    b. Continuous loop
    c. Shannon and Weaver communication model
    d. Berlo's communication process

143. Identify the patient statement that suggests the need for education:
    a. "I have a cataract growing on the outside of my eye."
    b. "I'm taking special vitamins to prevent macular degeneration."
    c. "I've been applying warm compresses to relieve a stye."
    d. "I have to change my contact lenses every day."

144. Your patient is a three-year-old girl. The shaft of her right humerus has a spiral fracture. She presents with numerous bruises on her arms, legs, and face, ranging from purple to yellow-green to brown. Her mother states her daughter fell off of a swing set while playing the previous evening. Your MOST appropriate action is to:
    a. Contact Child Protective Services within 24 hours
    b. Caution the mother to supervise the child during play
    c. Ask the child what happened
    d. Tell the mother you suspect child abuse

145. A mother believes her 6-year-old child has a hearing problem. Select the hearing test MOST appropriate for a school-aged child:
    a. Auditory brainstem response (ABR)
    b. Visual reinforcement audiometry (BRA)
    c. Conditioned play audiometry (CPA)
    d. Standard audiometry

146. Select the method that is NOT an example of secondary prevention (risk modification) for heart disease:
    a. An exercise program
    b. Diabetic management with a Hemoglobin A1c less than 7%
    c. Smoking cessation
    d. A lactose-free diet

147. Your patient is a 15-year-old boy. He has acute fever, chills, headache, confusion, hallucinations, photophobia, and nuchal rigidity. His Kernig and Brudzinski signs are positive. The MOST important diagnostic procedure is a:
    a. Complete blood count and differential
    b. Cranial MRI
    c. Lumbar puncture and examination of his cerebrospinal fluid
    d. Blood culture

148. A six-month old child should be able to:
    a. Roll over, roll from back to side, turn his head from any position, and sit with support for 10 to 15 minutes
    b. Sit alone, stand with support, and bounce on his legs
    c. Lift his head while prone or supine, turn from side to side, and roll stomach to back
    d. Crawl or creep readily, sit up, and pull himself up to a standing position

149. A principle of motivational interviewing techniques is to:
    a. Provide persuasion to elicit change
    b. Use constructive confrontation
    c. Maintain the role of expert
    d. Accept resistance to change

150. The World Health Organization states health promotion activities should focus on:
    a. The entire population
    b. The results of disease
    c. One primary method or approach
    d. Providing a medical service

Answer Key and Explanations

1. C: Allis' sign. An infant *older* than three months who holds one knee higher than the other during flexion (Allis' sign) has developmental hip dysplasia. The methods to assess an infant *younger* than three months are Barlow's test (pressing on the child's knees to pressurize the femoral head during hip flexion, causing posterior subluxation) and Ortolani test (rotating the child's hips through range-of-motion and listening for a click during abduction, as the femoral head slips). Adam's forward bending test is an assessment for scoliosis in children ages 10 to 15, which requires the child to bend over at the waist—as in toe touching—and the screener observes the hips to determine if there is a difference in height.

2. A: Provided subject to state restrictions and supervision requirements. Nurse Practitioners (NP) may bill Medicare for services in accordance with state restrictions and supervision requirements. The NP must bill using a National Provider Identification (NPI) number and meet the educational and licensing requirements for Nurse Practitioners. Some states require direct supervision by a physician *on the premises* while others require indirect or periodical supervision. The Centers for Medicare and Medicaid Services (CMS) pay for NP services that are: Medically necessary; equivalent to physician services; accurately documented on medical records; and billed correctly. Medicare may directly reimburse the NP, if state law allows it.

3. D: Renal failure. ACE inhibitors are contraindicated for patient with kidney failure, as one of their most serious side-effects is renal impairment, especially in patients who also take diuretics and NSAIDs. ACE inhibitors are commonly prescribed to treat hypertension and heart failure. They are often combined with diuretics, such as thiazide for hypertension or Lasix® for heart failure. ACE inhibitors are sometimes given to diabetics to prevent diabetic neuropathy.

4. B: Reasonable, measurable, and achievable. Patient-focused goal setting must be reasonable, measurable, and achievable. Patients are more motivated if they establish their own goals. The goals don't have to be simple, but they should be very specific, with short-term goals. Long-term goals may be the ultimate plan, but reaching long-term goals through a series of short-term goals is often more effective, because the patient is able to see progressive results. For example, losing weight in five-pound increments are easier short-term goals to achieve than the long-term goal of losing 50 pounds in total. Imbue your patient with confidence that the goals are achievable, to increase his/her motivation.

5. B: Hematocrit and hemoglobin to determine his blood loss. Order hematocrit and hemoglobin to determine if his blood loss is significant. Kiesselbach's plexus in the anterior nares has plentiful vessels and bleeds easily. Bleeding in the posterior nares is more dangerous and can result in considerable blood loss. Bleeding from the anterior nares is usually confined to one nostril. However, posterior nares bleeding may flow through both nostrils or backward into the throat, and the patient may be observed swallowing blood. Cocaine abusers suffer nosebleeds because of mucosal damage. Bleeding should stop within 20 minutes.

6. D: Advise her daughter that CPR must be withheld, in accordance with her mother's wishes. Explain to your patient's daughter that the health team cannot perform CPR because of the advance directive and desires of her mother. A valid DNR order is in place and does not require verification. Families often panic at the time of death and want life-saving measures, but this does not override the patient's explicit directions. The staff should provide emotional support for the family. While this is an ethical issue, there is no time to contact the Ethics Committee. Brain death occurs in 4 to 6 minutes.

7. C: Maintain an activity diary. Your patient should maintain an activity diary while wearing a Holter monitor, so any abnormality can be linked with the specific activity that triggered it. Conversely, the diary may demonstrate that no abnormality occurs with certain activities. Your patient should continue with prescribed medications and carry out normal activities, since the primary purpose of a Holter is to assist with diagnosis and to determine triggers for abnormal ECG readings. The monitor must be left on during the night, as some abnormalities occur during sleep, especially if the patient has sleep apnea.

8. D: Heart failure or left ventricular failure. The gallop rhythm is S3 occurring after S2. A gallop in older adults may indicate heart failure or left ventricular failure. A gallop may be a normal variant for children and young adults. An ejection click is a brief, high-pitched sound occurring immediately after S1, which occurs with aortic stenosis. An opening snap is an unusual, high-pitched sound after S2, which occurs with mitral stenosis from rheumatic heart disease. A friction rub is a harsh, grating sound heard in pericarditis. A heart murmur results from turbulent blood from stenotic or malfunctioning valves, congenital defects, or increased blood flow.

9. C: Practical and goal-oriented. According to Knowles, adult learners tend to be practical and goal-oriented, so they like to remain organized and keep the goal in mind while learning. Other characteristics of adult learners include:
- Self-directed: Adults like active involvement and responsibility
- Knowledgeable: Adults relate new material to familiar information gained through life experience or education
- Relevancy-oriented: Adults like to know how they will use new information
- Motivated: Adults like to see evidence of their own achievement, such as by gaining a certificate

10. D: Varenicline (Chantix®). Varenicline is a partial agonist of nicotinic acetylcholine receptors in the central nervous system. Close surveillance is required during therapy because Varenicline is one of the most potentially lethal drugs. The Institute for Safe Medication practices states Varenicline is responsible for seizures, cardiac arrhythmias, myocardial infarctions, diabetes, psychosis, aggression, suicide, severe skin reactions, serious accidents and falls, and aggression. Safer prescription medications to curb smoking are the nicotine inhaler, nicotine nasal spray, and bupropion (Zyban®). Bupropion can cause insomnia and dry mouth. OTC smoking cessation medications include nicotine gum, nicotine patches, and nicotine lozenges. These OTCs primarily cause local irritation.

11. C: Contracted service system. In contracted service, the Nurse Practitioner signs a contract and agrees to provide health care for a certain population, such as the homeless. The NP does not bill for individual services provided but is paid according to the contractual agreement. Fee-for-service reimbursement occurs when the patient pays the nurse directly

for services provided. Third-party reimbursement includes private insurance, Medicare, and Medicaid, which are billed for services provided to the patient. Third-party is the most common type of reimbursement. Second-party reimbursement occurs when a legal guardian/guarantor makes direct payment for services.

12. D: Health belief model. The health belief model predicts health behavior with the understanding that a person takes a health action to avoid negative consequences, if the person believes the action prevents negative outcomes. The theory is based on 6 basic perceptions:
- Susceptibility: Belief the person may develop a negative condition
- Severity: Understanding how serious a condition is
- Benefit: Belief that action reduces risk
- Barriers: Direct and psychological costs
- Action cues: Strategies, such as education, to encourage action
- Self-efficacy: Confidence in the ability to take action and to achieve positive results

13. C: All staff. All staff members are responsible for identifying performance improvement projects. Performance improvement must be a continuous process. Continuous Quality Improvement (CQI) is a management philosophy that emphasizes the organization's structure, and systems and processes within that organization, rather than individuals. Total Quality Management (TQM) is a management philosophy that espouses a commitment to meeting the needs of the customers (patients and staff) at all levels within an organization. Both management philosophies recognize that change can be made in small steps and should involve staff at all levels.

14. D: Refer him to a health agency that provides in-home care. Making a referral to a home health agency to provide in-home care is the best solutions, as this ensures that the man will receive skilled nursing care and still be able to stay at home with his grandson, who is too young for the responsibility of wound care. This is a more cost-effective solution than transferring the patient to an extended care facility. Keeping the patient in the hospital is not generally an option, as Medicare will not pay for extended care for long-term wound treatment.

15. A: Increased pressure in his right atrium and right heart failure. Increased jugular venous pressure (greater than 4 cm) indicates increased pressure in the patient's right atrium and right heart failure. It may also indicate pericarditis or tricuspid stenosis. Laughing or coughing may trigger the Valsalva response and also increase pressure. Jugular venous pressure is used to assess the cardiac output and pressure in the right heart, as the pulsations relate to changes in pressure in the right atrium. The jugular venous pressure is usually inaccurate if the patient's pulse rate exceeds 100 bpm. It is a non-invasive estimation of central venous pressure and waveform. Measure the internal jugular pressure, if possible; if not, the external jugular.

16. B: Thrombosis and vessel occlusion. Heparin-induced thrombocytopenia causes thrombosis syndrome. It puts the patient at increased risk for thrombosis and vessel occlusion, rather than hemorrhage. The drop in platelet count below 50,000 mm³ indicates this is type II, an auto immune reaction to heparin, rather than transient type I. Type II causes heparin-antibody complexes to form. The complexes release platelet factor 4, which in turn attracts heparin molecules that adhere to platelets and endothelial lining. The

misplaced heparin molecules stimulate thrombin and platelet clumping. Discontinue the heparin. Order treatment with direct thrombin inhibitors, such as lepirudin or argatroban.

17. C: He is in control of his health. A patient with an internal locus of control probably believes that he is in control of his health and that the actions he takes can make a significant difference. A patient with an internal locus of control prefers to participate in decision-making. A patient with an external locus of control is much more likely to believe that his health is related to bad luck or fate. A patient with an external locus of control prefers to leave decision-making and control in the hands of authorities, such as doctors and nurses.

18. C: Coarctation of the aorta. Coarctation of the aorta is a stricture of the aorta. The narrowing is proximal to the ductus arteriosus intersection. Blood pressure increases when the heart attempts to pump blood past the stricture. Strain causes the heart to enlarge. Blood pressure in the head and arms increases. Blood pressure in the lower trunk and legs decreases. With severe stricture, symptoms may not occur until the ductus arteriosus closes, causing sudden loss of blood supply to the lower body.

19. A: Check the laws for both states; complete two separate advance directives, each complying with one state's regulations. Explain to your patient that each state has its own unique regulations regarding advance directives. Direct your patient where to find both states' regulations. Obtain the proper forms, so your patient can complete two advance directives, if necessary. Most states require two witnesses, but some do not. Some states invalidate an advance directive if the author is a pregnant woman. It is inadequate for your patient merely to tell his family members his wishes. They may be unavailable during his cardiac arrest, or may be unwilling to carry out his wishes. Warn your patient not to store the advance directive in a safety deposit box, where access is limited to the key-holders.

20. C: Raise the heart rate between 80% and 90% of predicted for age and gender. The goal of the exercise stress test is to raise the patient's heart rate between 80% and 90% of predicted for age and gender. Cardiac stress testing determines if the coronary arteries dilate adequately during exercise. Normal coronary arteries dilate four times their resting diameter when under stress, so testing under exercise is more accurate to determine if there is compromised blood flow. The Bruce protocol, in which the speed and grade of the treadmill increases every 3 minutes, is most common. Chemical stress tests with adenosine or dipyridamole may be performed for patients who cannot tolerate exercise.

21. C: Group lecture and discussion. The most effective and efficient method for teaching lifestyle changes to a classroom of patients is the group lecture and discussion. This method allows the nurse to save time by providing the same information to all patients simultaneously, through a lecture. Afterward, patients share their concerns, interact, and discuss issues, which makes them feel engaged. Computer-assisted instruction is ineffective for some patients, especially groups of older adults. A lecture only is too passive and may not address the patients' concerns. One-on-one instruction is good for teaching specific processes or information, but is very time-consuming for the nurse. One-on-one instruction prevents patients from sharing their concerns with others, and can make individuals feel isolated.

22. B: Healthcare Common Procedure Coding System (HCPCS). CMS uses the Healthcare Common Procedure Coding System (HCPCS). HCPCS level I is based on CPT. Level II has

additional codes for supplies and services not covered by CPT. Current Procedure Terminology CPT, developed by the American Medical Association, provides codes for medical, surgical, and diagnostic services. International Statistical Classification of Diseases and Related Health Problems (ICD), developed by the World Health Organization, is used worldwide to identify conditions, including signs, symptoms, diseases, and traumatic injuries. ICD codes facilitate statistical studies of morbidity and mortality. Diagnosis-Related Group (DRG) classifies hospital cases into 500 to 600 groups, which have similar resource needs.

23. A: Digitalis toxicity. The most likely cause of these symptoms is digitalis toxicity. Most cases of digitalis toxicity can be traced to drug interactions. In this case, both furosemide and tetracycline can cause digitalis toxicity when taken with digoxin. Monitor your patient's digoxin levels at least monthly to ensure that therapeutic levels of 0.5 to 2.0 ng/mL are maintained. Early signs and symptoms of digitalis toxicity include fatigue, lethargy, depression, nausea and vomiting. Sudden changes in heart rhythm, AV or SA block, new ventricular dysrhythmias, and tachycardia may occur. Use digoxin immune FAB (Digibind®) to bind digoxin and inactivate it, if it climbs above therapeutic levels.

24. D: Tidal Volume. Tidal Volume (Vt) is the normal volume of air in one inhalation and exhalation, while the patient is at rest. Vt determines various lung volumes and capacities. Inspiratory reserve volume (IRV) is the amount of air inhaled during a forced inhalation, after a normal resting inspiratory effort. Expiratory reserve volume (ERV), conversely, is the amount of air exhaled through forced exhalation, after a normal resting exhalation. Residual volume (RV) is the volume of air remaining in the lungs after a forced exhalation.

25. D: A video. An adult-level video is an appropriate educational tool for an illiterate patient of normal intelligence. A children's book is inappropriate because your patient could feel infantilized. Third grade material is probably too difficult, especially if your patient is dyslexic. Even if your patient has some reading skills, third grade material may be too demanding and embarrassing during sickness and stress. Computerized instruction almost always involves some written instructions, so a computer is probably inappropriate. Allow your patient and his/her family to replay the video demonstration until they grasp the fundamentals well, before they must apply them. Videos are much more effective than written materials for those with low literacy or poor English skills.

26 C: The team leader who delegates the tasks. The nurse who delegates remains accountable for the patient outcomes and for supervision of the delegate. The scope of nursing includes delegation of tasks to unlicensed assistive personnel (UAP), such as school secretaries, providing those personnel have adequate training and knowledge. The nurse delegates to manage the workload and to provide adequate, safe care. Delegate in a manner that reduces liability. Provide adequate communication. The five rights of delegation are: Right task, right circumstance, right person, right direction, and right supervision.

27. A: Increase your caloric intake, exercise, and maintain your weight loss at 1 to 2 pounds per week. An 800-calorie per day diet is inadequate, and puts her body in starvation mode. The weight your patient lost so quickly will probably return just as quickly when she eats normally, as her body will now conserve fat. Your patient must increase her caloric intake, exercise 30 minutes daily, and maintain a slow weight loss of 1 to 2 pounds per week to keep it off long term. Advise your patient to maintain her exercise for at least 10 minutes at any one session. She does not need to sustain her effort for a full half hour session until she

builds up her endurance. Thirty minutes in total per day (10 min. X 3 sessions) is adequate. Refer this diabetic to a nutritionist to determine her best diet, rather than reducing calories independently.

28. A: Baseline drift. Baseline drift is an artifact resulting from poor contact between the electrodes and the patient's skin. Baseline drift often accompanies sweating (diaphoresis), or occurs when the patient wears heavy talc or body lotion. Baseline drift makes it difficult for the cardiologist to interpret the tracing. Gently clean the patient's skin. Apply extra electrolyte gel. Affix Micropore® tape over the electrodes to hold them steady and prevent baseline drift. Movement artifacts are the most common EKG problem, caused by muscle activity. Children and adult patients with movement disorders, chills, or anxiety have difficulty remaining still. Sixty Hz artifacts (electrical interference) occur when the EKG machine is near other electrical devices, such as monitors. Change the EKG plug to a green grounded electrical outlet. Use an alligator clip ground-wire. Move the electrical device temporarily, if it is safe to do so, to reduce interference.

29. B: Semiformal. Support systems provide both physical and emotional assistance. Semiformal support includes organizations and agencies in the community that provide goods or services. Semiformal support can be found at senior centers, religious and charitable organizations. Formal support is regulated by laws or statues. Formal social support is provided by social workers. Formal financial support is offered by Social Security and trusts. Formal medical support is provided by Medicare. Informal support derives from the social network. Informal support includes family and friends, but only those who actually provide assistance in some way. Support systems are critical for patients, especially isolated older adults. Patients without support turn to healthcare providers to fill their needs and may bond inappropriately.

30. A: An evidence review. An evidence review is the most important factor in developing evidence-based practices. Work systematically. First, review the literature at PubMed. Next, review best practices from the Agency for Healthcare Research and Quality and the Centre for Evidenced Based Medicine. Finally, write a critical analysis of these studies. Summarize the results, including pooled meta-analysis. Make your recommendations based on several recent expert opinions. You must have a minimum of two, written within the last five years. If there is inadequate evidence to review, rely on your personal experience and staff surveys. However, realize that anecdotal, subjective evidence is biased and is not a first-rate scientific source. Cost-effectiveness is an issue, but not your overriding concern.

31. D: Older Americans Act (OAA). The Older Americans Act (OAA) provides improved access to services for older adults and Native Americans, including community services (meals, transportation, home health care, adult day care, legal assistance, and home repair). The Emergency Medical Treatment and Active Labor Act (EMTALA) is designed to prevent patient "dumping" from Emergency Departments (premature discharge for economic reasons). The Omnibus Budget Reconciliation Act (OBRA) establishes guidelines for nursing facilities, such as long-term care facilities. The Americans with Disabilities Act (ADA) provides physically and mentally disabled patients access to employment and the community.

32. B: The right to pain control. The right to pain control is part of the Patients' Bill of Rights. Affordable healthcare and access to the latest medical technology are not included. The right to sue is not directly included, but patients are entitled to a procedure for registering

their complaints or grievances. Other provisions include: Respect for the patient; informed consent; advance directives and end-of-life care; privacy and confidentiality; protection from abuse and neglect; protection during research; appraisal of outcomes; appeal procedures; an organizational Code of Ethics; and formal procedures for donating and procuring organs and tissues.

33. B: Stop smoking. A person with Buerger's disease (thromboangiitis obliterans) should stop smoking immediately. Buerger's disease probably occurs from autoimmune dysfunction, resulting in recurrent inflammation of the small arteries and veins of the legs, and rarely the arms. Buerger's disease is non-atherosclerotic. It is most common in males, with onset between ages 20 to 35. It is virtually always associated with use of chewing or smoking tobacco. Treatment consists primarily of complete cessation of tobacco use, including exposure to second-hand smoke. Do not prescribe smoking cessation products that contain nicotine for Buerger's disease patients.

34. B: "Do you believe the treatment isn't helping you?" Demonstrate respect for your patient by asking a clear, direct, and polite question. Verbally express your message; do not merely imply it with body language or remain silent. Allow the child to explore how effective she perceives her treatment to be, and its likely outcomes. Never ignore the child's feelings. Elicit a response by stating, "I'd like to hear how you feel about that". However, you must still allow the child to terminate the discussion without further probing. Do not tell her simply, "Your parents decided about your treatment." Provide facts, but avoid using "should" or "must", because they often stop conversation. Deal with a child's issues immediately, rather than referring them to the doctor.

35. A: Autosomal recessive. People have 23 pairs of chromosomes. Half of each pair is inherited by the child from the father and the other half from the mother. Autosomal chromosomes are 1 through 22. X-linked and Y-linked disorders are related to chromosome pair 23. The autosomal recessive pattern of inheritance means both parents did not have an active form of Tay-Sachs disease, but they did each have a copy of the same abnormal gene on chromosome 15, which both passed along to their child. Every pregnancy presents the fetus with a 25% chance of inheriting fatal Tay-Sachs neurological damage, which usually causes death by age 4 or 5. The parents are carriers with a latent form of the disease, and their daughter suffers an active form of the disease. Autosomal dominant inheritance means one parent, with active disease, passes on an abnormal gene to the offspring.

36. D: Acupuncture. Acupuncture is traditional Chinese medicine (TCM). The practitioner inserts long, thin needles into trigger points along meridians. Acupuncture may reduce osteoarthritis and rheumatoid arthritis pain. Homeopathy is a German system based on the principal of like cures like. The practitioner dilutes miniscule doses of plants or minerals in water or alcohol to produce similar symptoms to the disease. Homeopathic healing is probably placebo effect. Aromatherapy uses essential oils from plant extracts. The practitioner applies oils topically to the patient's skin, or heats them for inhalation, or sprays the environment to treat and prevent disease. Orthomolecular therapy utilizes high doses of vitamins, minerals, amino acids, and essential fatty acids. The practitioner tries to nutritionally balance the patient, to counter environmental pollution and damage caused by processed foods.

37. A: A change in one person's behavior affects the others in the family. Bowen's family system theory considers the interdependence of family members, suggesting that a change

in one person's behavior will affect all the others. Bowen believes that family members vary in their need for external approval, but tend to function interdependently, even if they state otherwise. Triangle theory states the basic family unit is two people. When conflict arises, a third person is drawn into the conflict to provide stability by siding with one person or the other, maintaining the basic family unit.

38. C: Half of her sons and half of her daughters. A mother with an X-linked dominant disease can transmit the disease to 50% of her sons and 50% of her daughters. Males have only one X chromosome, so the male children will have a predictable disease. However, since female children have two X chromosomes, the normal X chromosome may compensate. Female symptoms of the disease vary from very minor to severe. If the father has an X-linked dominant disease, he passes the disease on to only his daughters. He inherited the abnormal gene from his own mother. His spouse provides the single X chromosome to her sons.

39. D: Immediately say, "The catheter was contaminated when it fell. Would you like me to get another setup or stay with the patient while you get it?" A contaminated catheter could cause septicemia. Advocate for the patient. Always prevent possible injury to a patient by interceding. First, state the problem simply: "The catheter was contaminated when it fell." Next, suggest a reasonable solution: "Would you like me to get another setup or stay with the patient?" Do not assign blame. Reporting the team leader's behavior to the supervisor is appropriate *after* protecting the patient. Do not leave the patient in danger while you fetch the supervisor. Saying nothing protects the team leader from possible repercussions, but is unprofessional conduct.

40. B: Five days. The girl should return in five days to have her sutures removed. Before prepping the tray for removal, consider the area involved, the circulation, and the degree of stress or pull on the wound. The face is a vascular area, so healing is usually faster than in other areas of the body, where sutures may remain in place for up to 10 days. In areas with increased stress, such as over joints, sutures may stay in place for even longer periods to ensure full thickness healing.

41. D: All of the above. The Health Insurance Portability and Accountability Act (HIPAA) addresses the rights of the individual and family to continue insurance after job loss or change, and to maintain the privacy of their health information. Personal or identifying information includes name, address, health history, diagnosis, and treatments in any form. Any electronic or paper documentation, or verbal communication, which contains the patient's personal or identifying information is considered protected health information (PHI). The entire healthcare team is required to protect its collection, storage, and transmission from theft, abuse, and prying eyes. HIPAA imposes national standards for electronic health records, and the Nurse Practitioner must work with the Medical Records and IT managers to comply.

42. D: The patient's behavior modification and compliance rates. Behavior modification and compliance rates are the best determinants of the effectiveness of patient education. Your patient may, indeed, be satisfied, may understand, and may be able to provide a demonstration. However, if your patient does not use what he learned, then your education of that patient was ineffective. Behavior modification involves thorough observation and measurement, identifying behavior that needs to be changed, and then planning and

instituting interventions. Determine the compliance rate by observation at intervals and on multiple occasions.

43. D: Rabies post-exposure prophylaxis (PEP). Many bats, foxes, raccoons, and skunks carry rabies. A lick or shallow puncture may transmit incurable rabies. Don PPE. Wash the bite wound. Inject 1 mL of PEP into the deltoid muscle of an adult, or anterolateral thigh for a child, on Day 0, and again on Day 3, 7, and 14 (4 doses in total). Give a fifth injection on Day 28, if your patient is immunosuppressed. Infiltrate 20 IU/kg of human rabies immune globulin (HRIG) into and around the bite wound on Day 0 only. If you cannot get the entire dose into the wound, inject the rest into a distant muscle with a clean needle. The process of twenty-three injections into the patient's abdomen was abandoned in the 1980s. Complete an animal bite report form. Fax it to your county's Public Health unit. Rabies incubation usually takes three to eight weeks. Rarely, it takes nine days or seven years. Watch for headache, fever, weakness, insomnia, anxiety, confusion, slight paralysis, agitation, hallucinations, hypersalivation, dysphagia, and hydrophobia.

44. C: Genetic predictive testing. Genetic predictive testing determines if the woman has the BRCA1 or BRCA2 gene associated with inherited breast cancers. Women carrying an abnormal gene have an 80% to 90% chance of developing breast or ovarian cancer. Ashkenazi Jews are high-risk. Mammograms prior to age 40 are inaccurate because young, dense breast tissue is difficult to map. Ultrasounds are more sensitive for dense breasts, but can indicate benign breast disease (BBD) that must be differentiated from cancer. Chest x-rays are ineffective for screening breast cancers. Thermography is a very sensitive, modern method for detecting tiny tumors.

45. A: A woman with advanced ovarian cancer. A woman with advanced ovarian cancer is NOT part of a vulnerable population because she can decide if research is in her best interests. Vulnerable populations are: Minor children (under 18); mentally incompetent patients; students and employees of research facilities; and prisoners. Explain your research to a child age 7 or older. Ask for his or her assent to participate. Include benefits, risks, alternative treatments, and the likely outcome of no treatment. The American Academy of Pediatrics states, "A patient's reluctance or refusal to assent should also carry considerable weight when the proposed intervention is not essential to his or her welfare and/or can be deferred without substantial risk." You must also obtain signed consent from the parents or guardian. It is illegal and unethical to manipulate patients and their parents to obtain sufficient subjects for your study. Consider that they may participate solely to gain privileges, so their self-reports may be skewed.

46. C: Bargaining. Grief is a normal response to a patient's abnormality, severe illness, or death. How a person deals with grief is very personal, and each will grieve differently. Elizabeth Kübler-Ross's five stages of grief are:
1. Denial: Resisting, not comprehending, or failing to remember information
2. Anger: Blaming self or others
3. Bargaining
4. Depression: Becoming tearful or withdrawn
5. Acceptance: Resolution

Bargaining involves if-then thinking. The patient and/or family may change doctors, thus trying to change the outcome, The patient and/or family may appeal to a deity, making promises such as, "I will go to church every day."

47. D: RICE (rest, ice, compress, elevate). RICE therapy (rest, ice, compress, elevate) is the primary treatment for Grade I, II and III sprains. Compress the injury with an elastic bandage or Aircast ankle brace to prevent swelling and to support the joint. Place ice in a plastic bag, then wrap it in a towel so that it does not cause frostbite. Ice the ankle for 20 minutes on and 20 minutes off to reduce pain and shrink injured vessels. Recline the patient and elevate the ankle above the heart level to reduce edema and promote circulation. Rest with minimal weight bearing and use of crutches for several days helps promote healing and prevents further damage.

48. C: Triglycerides. His triglycerides level should be less than 150 mg/dL. Your patient's blood triglycerides level is 50 mg/dL higher than normal range, which could contribute to pancreatitis. High triglyceride levels reflect his carbohydrate and alcohol intake, and increased stress. His LDL of 135 mg/dL is borderline; the optimal level is less than 100 mg/dL, and an acceptable range is 100 to 129 mg/dL. LDL reflects saturated fats in the diet. His HDL level of 55 mg/dL is near the optimal level of 60 mg/dL or higher. HDL below 40 mg/dL in males, or 50 mg/dL in females, increases the patient's risk of atherosclerosis and heart disease, because increased HDL protects against heart disease.

49. D: Bone scan. Stress fractures are common in runners and basketball players. A stress fracture is consistent with her symptoms. Stress fractures are hairline cracks that may not be evident on an x-ray. A bone scan may be necessary to diagnose a stress fracture. A tibial stress fracture may result from over-training, which is exercising beyond the patient's level of strength and endurance. Symptoms may be non-specific, but may involve point tenderness or increasing pain during activity, usually receding when at rest. Train her to use crutches, to reduce her weight bearing initially. Restrict her activities for up to three months to allow healing.

50. C: Provide opportunities for your patient to make decisions. Low self-esteem is common among older adults because they have to deal with so many losses. Seniors may become depressed, passive, and dependent. A good strategy for helping a senior overcome feelings of low self-esteem is providing opportunities for her to make independent decisions. Enhance your strategy by providing companionship, active listening, and encouraging your patient to express her feelings and concerns. Give positive feedback and praise only when she earns it, rather than praising everything she does. If you tell your patient she has no reason to be depressed, then you invalidate her feelings and further lower her self-esteem.

51. C: The individual state's Board of Nursing and *Nurse Practice Act*. The Nurse Practitioner's scope of practice is outlined by the state's Board of Nursing and *Nurse Practice Act*. A Registered Nurse who wants to become an Advanced Practice Nurse (APN) must first complete a Master's or doctoral degree (Ph.D.) at an accredited nursing school. Afterward, an advanced practice nurse must be accredited in a specialty by the American Nurses Credentialing Center (ANCC). Popular specialties include Family Nurse Practitioner (FNP), School Nursing, Home Health, and Perinatal Nursing. The American Nurses Association and the American Academy of Nurse Practitioners are professional organizations that help to set standards, but they do not have legal authority to determine the nurse's scope of practice.

52. B: Prospective payment system (PPS). A prospective payment system (PPS) pays a set amount for patient care, depending on the diagnosis-related group (DRG). A preferred provider organization (PPO) offers discounted rates to Medicare patients who choose their

healthcare providers from an authorized list. Listed providers agreed to accept Medicare assignment. Private insurance pay-for-service Medicare plans are contracted by Medicare. They provide more benefits, but the patient is required to work individually with the insurance company to determine benefits, and may be assessed an additionally monthly fee. Specialty plans are developed in different areas, many focusing on increased preventative care.

53. B: Increased protein. The average person requires about 0.8g of protein per kilogram of body weight every day (40 g to 70 g) to maintain good health. However, a burn patient needs more calories, minerals, vitamins, and protein than an average person, to ensure proper wound healing. If your burn patient is malnourished, then his wound healing will be delayed or complicated by edema. His burn will break open easily if his collagen is weak, and dietary protein is key for collagen synthesis. Increase the protein in your patient's diet to 1.25 g to 2.0 g per kilogram of body weight daily. Refer your patient to a dietician if he is concerned about calories, carbs, and fat because he is overweight. The dietician may supplement his diet with arginine, zinc, copper, iron, fatty acids, and Vitamins C, K, and B-complex while he is stressed by the burn.

54. A: Provide acceptance, and show no revulsion or negative feelings about your patient's appearance. A patient who experienced disfiguring surgery will predictably have a disturbed body image. Expect a period of adjustment before he attains self-acceptance. Telling your patient he is lucky to be recovering avoids the real issue. Use an interdisciplinary approach (Physiotherapy, Occupational Therapy, Psychology, Dietary, and Nursing), so he does not become dejected and dependent. He will probably feel depressed, disgusted, and may have phantom pain. He may refuse to participate in self-care initially, or even to look at his altered body part. Help your patient to dress in ways that minimize his exposure. Gently encourage him to touch and look at his altered body part. Persist in training him to perform self-care. Emphasize that he must stay well-groomed and odor-free.

55. A: Blood glucose and Hemoglobin A1c. His symptoms suggest diabetes mellitus type 2. Screen him with blood glucose and Hemoglobin A1c tests. Normal fasting blood glucose is less than 100 mg/dL and 2 hr. p.c. is less than 140 mg/dL. Pre-diabetic fasting glucose is 100 to 125 mg/dL and 2 hr. p.c. is 140 to 199 mg/dL. Diabetic fasting blood glucose is 126 mg/dL or more and 2 hr. p.c. is 200 mg/dL or more. Normal Hemoglobin A1c is 5% or less. Diabetic Hemoglobin A1c is ideally 6.5% to 7%. Diabetes correlates with obesity and race, especially in African Americans, Native Americans, Asians, and Hispanics. Obesity causes hypertension, hyperinsulinism, and insulin resistance. Diabetic children experience increased thirst, polyuria, and enuresis. Follow up with renal and thyroid tests if his screening is positive for diabetes. ECG is probably not indicated.

56. C: Skilled nursing facilities. An SNF provides both medical and personal care when a patient has problems with activities of daily living (ADL). A patient transfers to a SNF after an acute hospitalization, when the patient needs transitional care before returning home. An SNF patient needs more care than a home health agency or residential care facility can provide. An SNF patient is ineligible for a hospice, as she needs more than palliative care and is not dying. SNFs accept young adults and seniors who are mentally or physically disabled. Admissions range from a few days up to six weeks, depending on the patient's condition and progress. Most care is by certified nursing assistants, but SNFs usually provide some Physiotherapy, Occupational Therapy, Respiratory Therapy, Social Work and Recreation.

57. D: All females over age 21 or within 3 years of becoming sexually active. Screening for cervical cancer is recommended for all women no later than age 21, or within three years of their first sexual activity, whichever comes first. One-quarter of 15-year-olds have had two or more sexual partners. Therefore, start screening girls around age 16. Perform a pelvic exam with a Papanicolaou (Pap) smear. Talk to your patients ages 9 to 26 about Gardasil vaccine to prevent human papillomavirus (HPV, the most common sexually transmitted disease) and genital warts infections. Women age 30, or those with equivocal Pap results, need an HPV test to detect antibodies to HPV. A prior HPV infection increases your patient's risk of developing cervical cancer.

58. D: Cost comparisons. The AMA does not require cost comparisons as part of informed consent. Inform patients and their families about *all* their options. Allow their input on the type of treatments you offer, the reasonable risks, and any possible complications that are life-threatening or increase morbidity. All states require that you obtain informed consent, and the correct procedure is that you:
1. Explain the diagnosis
2. State the nature and reason for the treatment or procedure
3. List its risks and benefits
4. List alternative options (regardless of their cost or the patient's insurance coverage)
5. Outline the risks and benefits of alternative options
6. State the risks and benefits of declining a treatment or procedure (dissent)

59. A: Respect. In this case, averting her eyes is probably a sign of respect for you. A nurse is an authority figure. In many Asian cultures, it is considered disrespectful to look someone directly in the eyes for more than a quick glance. Prolonged eye contact is avoided because it is challenging or rude. The eyes are often averted downward to be polite. However, what is true for the group is not always true for the individual. The fact that the woman seems relaxed, rather than anxious, and is forthcoming with her responses, suggests that she is not fearful, depressed, or dishonest.

60. A: Cryotherapy. Cryotherapy is usually a spray of liquid nitrogen, but it may also be applied with a long cotton applicator (Q-tip) or a metal probe. Cryotherapy is an easy, effective, inexpensive remover of simple warts that works by necrosis when the cells freeze and thaw. Slight skin discoloration may occur, but it usually fades. Excision is more painful and carries an increased infection risk. Excision definitely results in a scar, so reserve it for more serious conditions, like skin cancer. A CO_2 laser often causes scarring, and is unnecessary for a small, single wart. Pulse dye lasers effectively remove warts, but are usually reserved for recurrent or multiple warts. Lasers are expensive for the Nurse Practitioner to acquire, and laser procedures are costly for the patient.

61. A: Medicaid. Medicaid is a combined federal and state welfare program authorized by Title XIX of the *Social Security Act* to assist low-income people of all ages with payments for medical care. Medicare, a federal health insurance program for those who have Social Security or have bought into Medicare, provides payment to private healthcare providers, such as physicians and hospitals, but limits reimbursement. Social Security is a federal pension program that provides old age, survivors, and disability insurance, with the monthly amount based on prior earnings. Supplemental Security Income (SSI), a federal program, provides additional money each month to seniors older than 65, the blind, or disabled people with low incomes and few resources.

62. C: Kinesthetic. Kinesthetic learners need to handle equipment, perform an action with minimal directions, and practice it independently to retain new information. They enjoy models blueprints, drawings, sculptures, dance, and working with their hands. They need to move and touch to learn. Let kinesthetic learners demonstrate their understanding by teaching the steps of the procedure back to you. Visual learners remember best by seeing flashcards, lists, videos, charts, diagrams, pictures, and demonstrations. They excel at sign language, spelling, and color. They have difficulty remembering names. Give them board notes, and quiet time to absorb written directions and manuals. Auditory learners are natural actors and may need to read aloud. They remember best through music, sound effects, and oral reports. They remember names and foreign languages well, but have difficulty with spoken directions. Auditory learners benefit from oral exams, audiotapes, group work, question periods, and discussions.

63. D: Complete a literature review. A literature review at The U.S. National Library of Medicine's PubMed is your first step in research. Before you formulate interview questions, check out the international Centre for Evidence Based Medicine. To create lists of possible causes and interventions, visit the U.S. Government's Agency for Healthcare Research and Quality. Follow these steps for a literature review:
1. Consider the source of the material (Web sites ending in .gov, .edu, and .org are best)
2. Review the author's credentials
3. Determine the author's thesis, or the central claim of the research, in the abstract
4. Examine the organization of the article
5. Review the evidence, including statistics and sample size (at least 500 is best)
6. Evaluate the article's overall credibility and usefulness

64. B: Her mother makes the decision, based on the *Durable Power of Attorney.* Your patient's mother has a legal document (PoA) granting her the authority to make healthcare decisions for her daughter, so she will make the decision about life support. Her daughter did not rescind the PoA, despite their estrangement, so there is no need to take the matter to court. Your patient's fiancé cannot make the decision because cohabiting does not confer legal authority. (Cohabiting is also a problem for gay and lesbian couples, who usually cannot legally marry, but may live as couples.) The father cannot make the decision because his legal custody ended when his daughter turned 18.

65. B: Aortic dilatation. This boy exhibits classic signs of Marfan syndrome. Screen him for aortic dilatation immediately, as he is at risk for a potentially fatal aortic dissection. Marfan syndrome is a genetic disorder of the connective tissue, related to protein metabolism. The tendons, ligaments, heart valves, and blood vessels of Marfan patients are often defective and weak. He may also suffer an aortic or mitral valve prolapse from connective tissue defects. When their connective tissue weakness is severe, restrict Marfan syndrome children from strenuous activities and team sports. Marfan children must especially avoid football and other contact sports that may result in chest trauma, or isometric exercises, such as weight lifting.

66. C: Dental. Phenytoin (Dilantin® and Epanutin) is only FDA-approved to control seizures. Its *off-label* uses are to control severe pain, mood disorders, high stress, and addictions. Primarily epileptics take phenytoin, but so do patients with sleep disorders, migraine, angina, post op pain, stroke pain, Sydenham muscle spasms, Parkinson disease, bullosa,

- 39 -

rheumatoid arthritis, AIDS, bulimia, alcoholism, and enuresis. Remind your patient who takes phenytoin to have regular dental examinations, because phenytoin causes gingival hyperplasia and bleeding gums. Hirsutism is a common side-effect, especially in dark women. Phenytoin also causes skin rash, nystagmus, vision disorders, dysrhythmias and dysarthria. Phenytoin taken in the first three months of pregnancy can cause mental retardation, slow growth, short fingers, and facial defects.

67. B: Your patient can list foods containing saturated and unsaturated fats. The learner outcome for teaching a patient with hyperlipidemia about diet should relate *directly* to that goal: List foods that contain saturated and unsaturated fats. Explaining the difference between LDL and HDL is important. However, lipid fractionation does not relate to the goal, and should not be the learner outcome for this activity. Advise your patients to use olive oil for cooking. Remind them to keep their triglyceride levels under 150 mg/dL. Your employer may require you to cover multiple dietary topics in one session, and achieve multiple outcomes. Beware of overwhelming frail patients with too much information.

68. A: Addison disease. These signs and symptoms are characteristic of Addison disease (primary adrenal insufficiency). Addison disease occurs when the adrenal cortex is damaged by autoimmune disease, genetic disorders, or destructive lesions or neoplasms. Without treatment, Addison disease is life-threatening. Be alert to bronze skin, profound fatigue, unexplained weight loss, weak muscles, and hypotension. Symptoms may be vague, so Addison disease is often undiagnosed until 80% to 90% of the adrenal cortex has been destroyed. Treatment is hormone replacement therapy with glucocorticoids (cortisol) and mineralocorticoids (aldosterone).

69. B: Meals-on-Wheels. Refer your patient to Meals-on-Wheels, to ensure adequate nutrition. This patient's poor vision and arthritis interfere with his ability to prepare meals. Home meal delivery programs provide low cost, nutritious meals for home-bound older adults. Your patient does not need care in an SNF, as his condition has stabilized. There is no indication for a referral to Medicaid because his eating choices relate to easy access, rather than lack of funds. Poor diet alone is not an indication for referral to Adult Protective Services.

70. A: Ask your patient to demonstrate for you. The best method to evaluate a patient's educational outcomes after you teach a procedure is to ask the patient to perform a demonstration. Your patient's verbal feedback is not a reliable indicator of his ability to perform independently. A pre-test is appropriate for determining your patient's existing knowledge about a specific subject, such as diet, so you can target your teaching to an appropriate level. Oral and written tests identify a patient's theoretical knowledge, but a passing mark does not ensure the patient can apply the practical skill. Remember that knowing and doing are different skills. Demonstration is critical, so the NP can provide feedback or additional training, if needed.

71. B: Airborne precautions. Airborne precautions protect the NP against small, suspended infectious agents that travel far from the patient on air currents, such as rubeola. An airborne infection isolation room must house a single patient, and it must have negative air pressure. All staff and visitors must wear respirators rated N95 or higher. Droplet precautions are for infectious agents with larger droplets that fall about three feet from the sneezing patient, such as meningococcal meningitis. Droplet precautions require private rooms or cohorting with more than three feet between beds and a separating curtain. Teach

- 40 -

your patient cough etiquette. Wear a mask when providing care. Use standard precautions for ALL patients. Follow hand hygiene, cough etiquette, safe injections, and use a mask for spinal or lumbar procedures. Contact precautions are for organisms spread by contact, such as *Clostridium difficile*. Don gown and gloves for care. House your patient in a separate room, or cohort multiple patients more than three feet apart.

72. C: Affordable Care Act. *The Affordable Care Act* of 2010 allows parents to keep their children on their health insurance policies until age 26. Another important provision prevents insurance companies from limiting or denying coverage for children younger than 19 with pre-existing medical conditions. The *Act* disallows lifetime dollar limits for care, prevents retroactive cancellation of policies because of mistakes on insurance applications without proof of fraud, and provides for an appeals process if claims are denied. Patients are allowed to choose their primary care physicians and pediatricians, to consult an OB-GYN specialist without referral, to use the nearest hospital Emergency Room, and to receive preventive services (such as vaccinations) at no cost.

73. D: Herpes zoster. Since 2006, the herpes zoster vaccine has been recommended for patients 60 years and older. It reduces the incidence of shingles by 50%. Hepatitis A vaccine is recommended for: One-year-olds; travelers; homosexuals; drug addicts; new adoptive parents of foreign babies; lab workers; patients with chronic liver disease; and patients receiving clotting factor concentrates. Hepatitis B vaccine is now recommended for newborns and older adults at risk of infection. Pneumococcal polysaccharide-23 vaccine (PPV, Pneumovax® and Pnu-Immune®) is now routinely given to Native Americans, children, seniors over 65, immunosuppressed and chronic patients (e.g., Hodgkin lymphoma, leukemia, AIDS, ESRD, asplenics, transplant recipients, alcoholics, anemics, and asthmatics).

74. C: Thyroid function tests. She has classic symptoms of hypothyroidism. Lithium increases her risk of developing thyroid disease because it inhibits her release of thyroid hormone. Order T3, T4, and TSH. Assess her other risk factors, such as iodine deficiency, radiation exposure, and aggressive treatment for goiter. Some dementia may occur with advanced thyroid conditions. Monitor her cholesterol, as it may increase and result in associated atherosclerosis and coronary artery disease. If her thyroid stimulating hormone (TSH or thyrotropin) level is below the normal reference range (usually 1 to 4 μU/mL, but depends on the testing laboratory), initiate daily treatment with synthetic levothyroxine (Synthroid®).

75. C: "You are shaking and seem worried." Simply acknowledge what is true and evident. Leave an opening for your patient to discuss his feelings. "What's wrong?" requires a direct response that your patient may not feel like giving immediately after a shock. "Do you want me to call your family?" does not deal with your patient's anxiety and is an escape for the nurse. "You don't need to worry. Everything will be all right," is a platitude that has little meaning and may not be true.

76. A: Human papillomavirus vaccine (Gardasil®). Human papillomavirus vaccine (Cervarix® or Gardasil®) is recommended for all females between the ages of 11 and 12 (although it may be given as early as age 9 for high-risk girls). Gardasil® is also given to males between 9 and 26 to prevent infection with genital warts. (Cervarix® does not confer genital wart protection.) Rotavirus vaccine prevents severe rotavirus-related diarrhea and is given to babies in three separate doses (2 months, 4 months, and 6 months). Hepatitis A

vaccine is given to toddlers in two separate doses (12 months and 18 months). Measles, mumps, and rubella (MMR) vaccine is given in two separate doses (12 to 18 months and 4 to 6 years).

77. B: Healthcare-associated infection. According to the CDC (2007), healthcare-associated infections are all infections related to healthcare, whether in an acute setting, such as a hospital, a clinic, or a skilled nursing facility, or in the home. This broad term reflects the difficulty presented to Infection Control in pinpointing at which point or place in treatment an infection arises. For example, a patient may contract an infection in the hospital, but is asymptomatic at discharge, and symptoms present at home. The term nosocomial infection now refers specifically to an infection that is acquired during hospitalization. Community-associated infections are acquired by people who had no contact with healthcare workers, usually for more than year.

78. D: Marked hypotension and anuria, in addition to other symptoms. Dehydration results from: Inadequate fluid intake, often because mouth sores or laryngitis deter drinking; excess water loss from sweating during heavy exercise; aggressive NG suctioning; excessive diuretic drugs; diarrhea and vomiting; uncontrolled diabetes; and fever. Mild dehydration is a 5% loss of body fluid, characterized by: Dizziness; lethargy; reduced skin turgor; dry mucous membranes; dark yellow urine; and orthostatic hypotension. Moderate dehydration is a 10% loss of body fluid, characterized by: Confusion; resting hypotension; tachycardia; and oliguria or anuria. Severe dehydration is fluid loss exceeding 15%. Severe dehydration occurs when total body water decreases but sodium does not. It is characterized by: Marked hypotension; anuria; sunken, tearless eyes; sunken fontanelles in babies; dry, sticky mouth; delayed capillary refill; lethargy progressing to shock and coma.

79. D: Both verbal and non-verbal responses. Both your patient's verbal and non-verbal responses may be of equal importance. If your patient looks away or becomes tense, it could mean he is not telling the truth or does not want to answer. However, you must take into account cultural norms if your patient is not American-born. The information you elicit during an interview should include not only the patient's medical facts, but also his attitudes and concerns, because they impact his compliance. Ask open-ended questions, rather than closed questions that elicit only yes/no responses. Ask clarifying questions if the response is ambiguous. Provide a list of options. Employ active listening by rephrasing your patient's statement to encourage him to elaborate more.

80. B: Pharmacodynamics. Pharmacodynamics relates to the biological effects (therapeutic or adverse) of drug administration over time. You must consider the method of drug transport, absorption rate, means of elimination, and drug half-life. Pharmacokinetics relates to the effect the body has on the drug, considering the route of administration, the absorption rate, the dosage, the frequency of administration, the distribution, and the serum levels achieved over time. Half-time is the time needed to reduce plasma concentrations to 50% during elimination. Usually, the equivalent of 5 half-times is needed to completely eliminate a drug or achieve steady-state plasma concentrations, if you dose the patient intermittently. Effect-site equilibrium is the time between your administration of a drug and its clinical effect.

81. D: Clinical decision support systems (CDSS). CDSS are interactive software applications that help you to make healthcare decisions. The applications contain a database of medical knowledge. You enter patient data. An evidence-based inference system provides patient-

specific advice. Computerized physician/provider order entry (CPOE) is a clinical software application that automates medication and treatment ordering. CPOE must be typed in a standardized format to avoid mistakes. The computerized notification system provides alerts related to abnormal laboratory or imaging results. The Electronic medical record (EMR) is a digital computerized patient record, which may be integrated with CPOE and CDSS to improve patient care and reduce medical errors.

82. B: Echocardiogram. An echo shows the functioning of the patient's heart valves, blood flow through the heart, and measures the ejection fraction (percentage of blood pumped from the left ventricle during each contraction). The ejection fraction is usually normal if the patient has diastolic failure. Patients with systolic failure have less than 40% ejection fraction because the heart cannot pump adequately. A chest x-ray shows enlargement of the heart (cardiomegaly) and pulmonary edema. An angiogram shows blood circulation, especially through the coronary arteries, indicating areas of obstruction. An EKG indicates heart rate and rhythm, to identify arrhythmias and previous cardiac damage.

83. C: Arrange for a professional translator to attend the intake. Book a qualified translator ahead of time. Do not rely on support staff who speak the foreign language but lack medical terminology. Never use a minor as a translator because it is not an age-appropriate responsibility. Children lack the necessary vocabulary and understanding about health matters. In some cultures, it is rude to tell a sick person directly about a serious illness, so the child may not interpret correctly. Unless your patient is unable to answer questions independently because of his health condition, do not ask his wife or another adult relative to answer questions for him. Proxy answers violate his confidentiality. He may not honestly answer you about sexual history and other sensitive questions with family present. They may not understand medical terminology and may translate incorrectly.

84. D: *Clostridium difficile.* The CDC recommends contact precautions for *Clostridium difficile,* which is spread by fecal contamination. Antibiotic-resistant *Clostridium difficile* is a growing threat to hospitalized patients. Other agents requiring contact precautions include VRE and RSV. Hepatitis B requires standard precautions. *Mycobacterium tuberculosis,* rubeola (measles) and varicella (chickenpox) require airborne precautions because their droplets are airborne and spread over long distances (more than three feet from the patient). *Haemophilus influenzae, Neisseria meningitidis, Group A Streptococcus, and B. pertussis* require droplet precautions because they usually spread less than three feet from the patient after a sneeze or cough.

85. A: Functional urinary incontinence. Functional incontinence means the patient cannot make it to the bathroom in time, due to slow movement, poor cognition, or miscommunication. It happens frequently to patients with Alzheimer and Parkinson diseases, and arthritis. Stress incontinence occurs in mothers, menopausal women with dry mucosa, and men with prostate enlargement. Their weakened pelvic muscles allow small squirts of urine to leak involuntarily during sneezing, laughing, coughing, exercising, standing abruptly, and lifting weights. Overflow incontinence means the bladder is constantly distended. It happens with: Diabetic neuropathy; calculi; prostatic hypertrophy; tumors; birth defects; and tight bladder surgery. Urge incontinence is spastic bladder from irritation. It occurs with: A bladder infection; interstitial cystitis; tumors in the prostate, uterus, or bladder; Parkinson or Alzheimer diseases; stroke; hysterectomy; prostatitis; multiple sclerosis; caesarean section; or pelvic surgery. The patient urinates more than

- 43 -

seven times daily, or twice nightly. The patient has a sudden, reflexive urge to urinate when hearing running water, drinking, or sleeping.

86. C: Gluten free. A gluten-free diet is necessary to treat celiac disease (sprue), which is an autoimmune disorder. The celiac patient cannot tolerate gluten in barley, rye or wheat bread. Many cosmetics, drugs, and vitamins contain gluten as a binder. Celiac disease destroys surface epithelium in the small intestine. Signs and symptoms include: Abdominal bloating and colic; weight loss due to impaired absorption; diarrhea; bloating; steatorrhea (fatty stools); azotorrhea (excessive nitrogen loss); and anemia due to iron, Vitamin B_{12}, and folate deficiencies. Steatorrhea occurs because digestion of fats is impaired, but a low fat/low carbohydrate diet will not relieve the celiac patient's symptoms. Lactose free diets are for those with lactose intolerance.

87. B: Preoperational. According to Piaget's theory of cognitive development, children engage in magical thinking and show egocentrism in the preoperational stage. Piaget's four stages are:
1. Sensorimotor (0-24 months): Intellect begins to develop. Children acquire motor and reasoning skills, begin to use language, and prepare for more complex intellectual activities.
2. Preoperational (2-7 years): Children develop a beginning concept of cause and effect, along with magical thinking and egocentrism.
3. Concrete operations (7-11): Children develop understanding of cause and effect with regard to concrete thinking. They cannot think abstractly.
4. Formal operational (11-adult): Children/young adults develop mature though processes, the ability to think abstractly, and to evaluate different possibilities and outcomes.

88. B: Mini-cog test. The Mini-cog test assesses dementia. The NP asks the patient to remember and repeat back three common objects. The patient draws a clock face indicating a particular time. MMSE assesses dementia through a series of tests, including remembering the names of three common objects, counting backward, naming, providing location, copying shapes, and following directions. The Digit Repetition Test assesses attention by asking the patient to repeat two numbers, then three, then four, and so on. The Confusion Assessment Method is used to assess delirium, not dementia.

89. C: Thiazide diuretic. Long-acting thiazide diuretics (such as chlorothiazide and chlorthalidone) are the first-line treatment for mild hypertension. Thiazides inhibit reabsorption of sodium and chloride. They force the urinary system to excrete more sodium, potassium, bicarbonate, and water. Hence, thiazides are given with potassium, or in combination with potassium-sparing diuretics, such as spironolactone or eplerenone. Potassium-sparing diuretics may cause hyperkalemia if given alone. Loop diuretics, such as furosemide and bumetanide, increase excretion of sodium, chloride and other electrolytes, so they may cause electrolyte imbalances. Loop diuretics are short-acting and less effective for treating hypertension.

90. D: Use a clean needle and clean syringe for each of the three drugs. The CDC guidelines for safe injections state that a clean needle and syringe should be used for *every* injection to avoid contamination. Avoid multiple dose vials, because each needle insertion increases the danger of contamination. The CDC traced outbreaks to healthcare workers reinserting

needles into multi-dose vials or IV bags, and then using the same needle and syringe to give IV drugs to more than one patient. In some cases, the contamination occurred when healthcare workers prepared medications in Dirty Utility rooms (areas where used needles and syringes are broken and disposed of in Sharps containers). Prepare medications only in the designated Pharmacy area or Clean Utility room on your unit.

91. B: Bandura's theory of social learning. Bandura proposed that children learn from interacting with adults and through modeling behavior. Kohlberg's theory of moral development outlines the three progressive stages in which children learn a sense of morality: Preconventional, conventional, and postconventional. Watson's theory of behaviorism uses the concept of positive reinforcement, and suggests children can be controlled by proper application or withholding of rewards. Chess and Thomas's temperament theory uses nine personality parameters to describe children's response to events. It differentiates the difficult child, slow-to-warm-up child, and easy child.

92. A: Immediately. For legal reasons, the NP must always document medication administration, vital signs, interventions, and changes in condition immediately. Document routine care in the patient's chart every 1 to 2 hours. Routine care includes assisting with activities of daily living, such as bathing, ambulation, dressing, feeding, and toileting. Failure to chart medications in a timely manner may result in your patient receiving the medication twice. Overdoses are especially common after shift change. When one nurse cares for several patients, it is easy to forget, omit, or confuse information. Charting in advance is always illegal and dangerous because it can lead to medication errors. Never assume that a client will have no problems on your shift. If you chart routine care previous to performing the acts, it can result in time-consuming corrections.

93. A: Order sputum culture and sensitivities. Bronchitis is inflammation of the trachea and bronchi (tracheobronchial tree). It often occurs as a progression of an upper respiratory infection. Bronchitis is usually caused by viruses, but can also be caused by bacteria and fungi. Viral bronchitis is usually a mild, self-limiting disorder characterized by a dry, hacking cough that tends to worsen at night and is productive within 2 or 3 days of onset. It generally clears within 5 to 10 days. Bronchitis that persists for longer than 10 days may not be viral. Order sputum for C&S prior to prescribing antibiotics.

94. A: Hyperkalemia. Normal blood potassium ranges from 3 to 5 mEq/L and requires a daily dietary intake of 70 to 100 mEq/L. Hyperkalemia is excessive blood potassium (more than 5 mEq/L), which often occurs with renal disease. Hyperkalemia is characterized by ventricular arrhythmia, weakness, ascending paralysis, hyperreflexia, diarrhea, and confusion. Hypokalemia (blood potassium less than 3 mEq/L) is characterized by weakness, lethargy, nausea, vomiting, paresthesias, dysrhythmias (PVCs with flattened T-waves), muscle cramps with hyporeflexia, hypotension, and tetany. Normal blood calcium ranges from 8.5 to 10.2 mg/d Land requires a daily dietary intake of 1 g for adults. Hypocalcemia (less than 8.5 mg/dL) is characterized by tetany, tingling, seizures, altered mental status, and ventricular tachycardia. Hypercalcemia (more than 10.2 mg/dL) is characterized by increasing muscle weakness with hypotonicity, constipation, anorexia, nausea, vomiting, and bradycardia.

95. C: Close your patient's door to allow them privacy. Treat your patient holistically and with compassion. People of all ages need intimacy. Your patient is a mentally alert, consenting adult. Consider it a conjugal visit. The most appropriate action is to quietly and

unobtrusively close your patient's door to allow the couple privacy. It is wrong to assume that seniors have less need for intimacy than younger adults, or that expressions of intimacy are inappropriate in a hospital. While her husband should have thought to secure the door, embarrassing either or both of them serves little purpose. Asking her husband to leave is a form of punishment.

96. A: A daily stool softener, such as Colace®. A stool softener decreases fluid absorption in the bowel. It moves stool through the colon more quickly and can be administered daily. A bulk former, such as Metamucil®, may also be helpful, but fiber has already been added to her diet without relieving her constipation. Your patient should not take laxatives routinely because the bowel becomes dependent on them; in time, constipation worsens. Avoid routine enemas of any kind, unless absolutely necessary to relieve impaction as they may cause loss of muscle tone and irritation of the intestine.

97. C: Mobility and risk of falls. The timed-up-and-go (TUG) test assesses mobility and the risk of falls. The patient begins seated in a chair with armrests. The patient stands up, walks 3 meters, turns, and sits back down in the chair. The normal time to complete this sequence is 7 to 10 seconds. If the patient requires 14 seconds or longer, it mean he or she is at-risk for falls. The TUG-cognitive is a modified version that requires the patient to carry out the same sequence while counting backwards from a number between 20 and 100. The TUG-manual version requires the patient to carry out the sequence while carrying a cup full of water. The longer the time required for these tasks, the higher the fall risk, and the lower the patient's functional ability.

98. A: Cocaine. Your patient exhibits clear signs of cocaine abuse. His nasal irritation and nosebleeds indicate he snorts cocaine. His lip burns and cough indicates he smokes crack or freebases. Constricted pupils, headaches, and abdominal pain are common among cocaine abusers. Many drugs of abuse can produce similar symptoms. However, a heroin abuser has needle tracks and no nasal irritation. A heavy marijuana abuser might have tachycardia and cough from lung irritation (similar to tobacco smokers). However, marijuana abuse by itself rarely causes nasal irritation or nose bleeds. (A grow-op laden with mold spores could cause the URI symptoms.) Marijuana is more likely to cause mydriasis (pupils dilated more than 5 mm) and red eyes from vessel dilation. Methadone abuse constricts pupils (miosis, pupils shrunken to 2 mm or less) and creates abdominal pain, but does not cause nasal symptoms.

99. D: Provide full information to the parents, and allow them to express their feelings. *Adult* Jehovah's Witnesses often refuse whole blood, packed red cells, white cells, or plasma for their personal health. However, parents may allow their children to receive minor blood products (fractionated cells and hemoglobin-based blood substitutes) if the hemoglobin drops below 10 g/dL. Your FIRST step is to approach the parents empathetically and explain their son's dire need for a blood transfusion or blood components. Give them full information without being judgmental. Allow them to express their feelings. Jehovah's Witnesses allow synthetic (recombinant) erythropoietin (EPO) and blood expanders, such as saline, Hetastarch (HES), dextran, lactated Ringer's solution, and Hemaccel. They also permit surgeons to slow bleeding by cooling the patient, hypotensive anesthesia, and Desmopressin (DDAVP). Never assume that religious beliefs alone determine parent's actions; they are concerned about HIV and hepatitis.

100. A: Discontinue lithium until her blood level is less than 1.5 mEq/L. Stop her lithium immediately. The normal therapeutic range is 0.6 to 1.2 mEq/L for adults. The effective dose is very close to the toxic dose (narrow therapeutic index). Mild lithium toxicity (1.5 to 2.5 mEq/L) produces severe vomiting, diarrhea, increased muscle tremors and twitching, lethargy, body aches, ataxia, tinnitus, blurred vision, vertigo, and hyperactive deep tendon reflexes. Severe lithium toxicity (2.5 mEq/L and above) produces fever, oliguria (less than 500 ml of urine in 24 hours), hypotension, EKG abnormalities, decreased level of consciousness, seizures, coma, and death. Order electrolytes, anion gap, renal function tests, routine urinalysis with specific gravity (SG), and an EKG. Plasma levels usually decrease to the normal range within 48 hours after discontinuing lithium. Lithium does not bind to charcoal, but a doctor can perform whole-bowel lavage with polyethylene glycol, and order hemodialysis.

101. B: The integration of nursing, computer, and information sciences in the management of data and information. Nursing informatics is the integration of nursing, computer, and information sciences in the management of data and information. Informatics seeks methods to streamline and improve documenting data and managing information. Nursing informatics involves research into the best systems and evaluation of existing systems. ANCC provides credentialing for nurse informatics specialists, requiring specific coursework. Nurse informatics specialists are involved in system design and often have a pivotal role in improving patient safety and facilitating user education. They facilitate the use of smart technology, wireless remote monitoring, and electronic record keeping.

102. B: Monoamine oxidase inhibitors. Combining an SSRI with a MAOI may result in serotonin syndrome, a potentially life-threatening disorder. The SSRI and NSAID combination increases the patient's risk of upper GI bleeding, although the risk is lessened with the addition of acid-suppressing medication. When an SSRI is combined with digoxin, the blood level of digoxin may increase, leading to digitalis toxicity. Combining an SSRI with alcohol can increase drowsiness and craving for alcohol, which increases the patient's risk of alcoholism.

103. C: Educate her about birth control methods. The rhythm method is unreliable. Even strict adherence to the Billings Ovulation method of monitoring cervical mucus, temperature, and calendar, with Early Days and Peak rules, has a failure rate of 4%. Advising total abstinence is unrealistic. Teach the girl about superior birth control methods. Emphasize the use of barrier contraceptives, such as condoms, which also protect against sexually transmitted diseases. Telling the girl's parents would violate confidentiality. Sexual activity alone is not a reason to refer a girl to counseling, as almost half of teenagers between 15 and 18 are sexually active.

104. D: State you cannot do so personally, but will help her to call a friend or family member. While gathering the materials may benefit your patient in the short term, unwanted transference may occur. You do not want to establish a relationship of increasing dependency and obligation that does not resolve the long-term needs of your patient. Offer to help by calling a friend or family member to bring them to her. Since your patient is quite ill and may have difficulty making other arrangements, simply refusing and citing policy (while true) ignores your patient's needs. Asking another person (manager) to do so would never be appropriate because it violates confidentiality.

105. A: Aching, cramping leg pain; brownish discoloration of his ankles and shin (anterior tibia). Peripheral *venous* insufficiency is characterized by aching, cramping leg pain, present pulses, brownish discoloration around the ankles and anterior tibial area, and moderate to severe edema. Superficial, irregular, ulcers may appear on the medial or lateral malleolus, and/or anterior tibial area.

106. B: Observe her breastfeeding and educate her about correct infant positioning and latching on. Breastfeeding pain is almost always caused by improper infant positioning or incorrect positioning of the mouth about the nipple and areola. Watch the mother's breastfeeding technique and gently correct it. Mothers were advised to "toughen" their nipples until the 1970s, but rough handling causes tiny cracks that invite mastitis. Mothers should not experience pain, but just a let-down reflex. Sometimes, trouble latching on occurs if the nipples are too small or too large, but changing position helps. Flat or inverted nipples usually begin to elongate within a few minutes of stimulation. Avoid nipple shields, as they prevent the breast from getting adequate stimulation and require the infant to work harder for less milk.

107. B: Post-traumatic stress disorder. PTSD is a response to a severe emotional or physical trauma. PTSD is one of the anxiety disorders. The patient is typically numb after the initial trauma. Later, after survival is no longer an issue, the patient develops excessive irritability, nightmares, flashbacks to the traumatic scene, and overreactions to sudden noises and movements. PTSD typically develops after a terrifying ordeal that involved physical harm or the threat of physical harm, such as military combat, assault, rape, serious accidents, abuse, and natural disasters.

108. B: Driver. Drivers are opinionated, decisive, and demand results. They like to be in charge and may respond to stress by becoming demanding. Drivers try to control their lives. Expressors get excited and show concern about who is providing services, but are less interested in facts and details than drivers. The expressor's reaction to stress is to press their own ideas, or to become argumentative. Relaters like to be helpful and positive. Relaters want to understand the reasons for things. Under stress, they are more likely to become withdrawn. Analyticals focus on data. They are very methodical and ask technical questions about how things work. Under pressure, analyticals tend to seek even more information.

109. C: Hand express her milk, and massage the breast lump under a warm shower. Encourage her to open her blocked milk ducts by hand expressing milk and massaging the lump under a warm shower. Avoiding breastfeeding will worsen the condition because the breasts become engorged. If the blockage persists more than 48 hours, therapeutic ultrasound (2 watts/cm^2) for 5 minutes may reduce the blockage. Do not prescribe antibiotics unless the blockage persists and mastitis develops. Advise the mother to continue frequent breastfeeding on both sides, while massaging the blocked area. Warm (not hot) compresses may also provide some relief, but ice packs should not be applied. The mother should vary the infant's position when nursing, to ensure the entire breast is drained. Teach her the football hold.

110. A: Intimacy vs. isolation. The conflict associated with young adulthood is intimacy versus isolation, which can lead to lack of close relationship or love and intimacy. Erikson's 8 stages include five related to childhood and three related to adulthood:

1. Trust vs. mistrust: Birth to 1 year
2. Autonomy vs. shame/doubt: 1 to 3 years
3. Initiative vs. guilt: 3 to 6 years
4. Industry vs. inferiority: 6 to 12 years
5. Identity vs. role confusion: 12 to 18 years
6. Intimacy vs. isolation: Young adulthood
7. Generativity vs. stagnation: Middle age
8. Ego integrity vs. despair: Older adulthood

111. C: Draw one ink line through the charting error, write "Error" above it, and initial and date your change. A charting error must be acknowledged by drawing a line through the text and writing "Error." Remember that the patient's chart is a legal document, subpoenable to court. Since a judge, police, and lawyers may examine your notes, you cannot erase it or make it illegible with strike-overs or correction tape or fluid. Providing an extended explanation is unnecessary for most charting errors. However, if the medication has already been administered to the wrong patient, then the drug error must be indicated in the patient's chart, and you must also prepare a separate incident report form. Incident report forms go to the unit supervisor and Risk Manager, and are not included as part of the patient's record.

112. B: Speak slowly and clearly, and let the patient use a picture chart to respond. People with Broca's (non-fluent) aphasia can usually understand speech fairly well if you speak slowly and clearly. Aphasia patients who have trouble responding use truncated phrases instead of whole sentences, such as, "water, water" instead of "I'd like water." Picture charts can help them respond. Wernicke's (fluent) aphasia from damage to the temporal lobe causes difficulty understanding language. However, a Wernicke's patient retains the ability to understand gestures and produce some language. Patients may be able to write or use letter boards. Global (non-fluent) aphasia results from extensive damage to language centers. Global aphasia causes difficulty with both understanding and producing language, so pictures, diagrams, picture charts, and gestures are helpful.

113. B: Splint his arm securely, without attempting to change the degree of flexion. Splint his arm to maintain its position and relieve muscle spasms. You may also apply a sling to maintain bone alignment, providing he can tolerate the movement, but do not attempt further treatment until your patient has an x-ray to determine the extent of his injury. If you change its flexion, put the arm though range-of-motion exercises, or apply a compression dressing, you may cause severe pain and additional damage to the joint. The radiologist must determine whether your patient's elbow is fractured or dislocated, and the degree of injury. Displaced fractures may require open reduction by an orthopedic surgeon.

114. D: Mesothelioma. Mesothelioma is cancer of the mesothelial cells found in organ linings such as the pleura. Ninety percent of mesotheliomas occur in the lungs. The malignancy may metastasize to adjoining tissues. Mesothelioma is associated with exposure to asbestos, a product used in construction until the late 1970s as a fire retardant. Mesothelioma has a delayed onset, so symptoms usually appear between ages 50 and 70, primarily in males. Unlike other types of lung cancers, mesothelioma is *not* associated with smoking; it is usually a work-related injury. Asthma and COPD are not usually associated with chronic pain.

115. C: Orlistat (Xenical®, Alli®). Orlistat helps reduce weight by preventing absorption of fat. It inhibits the pancreatic and gastric enzymes that break triglycerides into fatty acids, so fats pass into the stool. It also inhibits absorption of fat-soluble vitamins (A, D, E and K). Benzphetamine and diethylpropion are central nervous system stimulants, which decrease appetite, but may be habit-forming. Phentermine is an appetite suppressant that reduces hunger by increasing the adrenals' production of norepinephrine. Medications should be supervised and reserved for obese patients with a BMI greater than 30, or for overweight patients with a BMI greater than 27 who have associated health risks, such as hypertension or diabetes.

116. D: Insist on telling her parents with the girl present; support the girl and help the family to discuss the issue. The nurse practitioner is often faced with ethical concerns regarding confidentiality for mature minors. Different ethics apply to birth control and mental health. Deal with the issue directly by informing the adolescent *before treatment begins* that what she says will be held in confidence *within certain limitations.* She reaches the limit when she becomes a threat to self or others. Health endangerment through alcohol or drug abuse, eating disorders, or suicidal ideation must be reported to her parents because they are potentially life-threatening. Assure the adolescent that you will be present to support her when she discusses these matters with her parents. Uphold your mandatory reporting requirements by reporting to the proper authorities within 24 hours incidents of child abuse, sexual abuse, and communicable diseases.

117. C: "Are you in immediate danger, and is your abuser on the premises?" Females are the most common victims of domestic violence, but there are increasing reports from male victims, both in heterosexual and homosexual relationships. Your patient's immediate safety is always the most important consideration in domestic violence situations. First, determine if your patient is in immediate danger and if his abuser is on the premises. Your patient's abusive partner could pose a threat to both your patient and you, the intervenor. When you are certain you do not need to vacate the premises, ensure they are secure. Obtain a complete history of the types and patterns of your patient's abuse. Provide him with information and a list of shelter resources. Avoid providing "should" advice to patients who are already frightened and intimidated.

118. B: Pernicious anemia (Vitamin B_{12}/cobalamin deficiency). Pernicious anemia is a megaloblastic anemia resulting from cobalamin (Vitamin B_{12}) deficiency. Pernicious anemia is common among the following types of patients: Seniors older than 50; post-op gastric surgery; post-op ileectomy; Crohn's disease; long-term users of H_2-histamine receptor blockers (which reduces hydrochloric acid); strict vegetarians for more than five years. Intrinsic factor (IF) is a carrier protein normally produced by parietal cells of the gastric mucosa. Patients with pernicious anemia lack IF because of atrophy or autoimmune destruction of their parietal cells, which also decreases their hydrochloric acid secretion. Hydrochloric acid is necessary for secretion of IF, and IF is necessary for cobalamin absorption.

119. C: 10 to 15 psi. Wound irrigation pressures should be 10 to 15 psi for effective cleaning. Pressure less than 4 psi is inadequate to clean a wound properly. Pressures between 4 and 9 psi provide weak cleansing only, but may be appropriate for exposed blood vessels or graft sites, when you must avoid sloughing skin. A 250 mL squeeze bottle provides irrigation at 4.5 psi. Bulb syringes are portable, but less effective than mechanical irrigation devices. Pulsed lavage is usually set between 8 and 15 psi. A 35 cc syringe topped

- 50 -

with a 19-gauge needle provides irrigation at 8 psi. Pressure greater than 15 psi increases wound trauma.

120. D: Financial abuse. Financial abuse includes: Theft; coercion to give away or sign away belongings; convincing the victim to invest in fraudulent schemes or change provisions of her Will; and moving permanently into the victim's home, taking it over without sharing costs. Neglect may be active, from lack of caring, or passive, from inability to provide adequate care. Physical abuse is active and includes hitting, biting, pulling hair, and shoving. Psychological abuse includes threats, intimidation, and forced seclusion. Sexual abuse is also a common danger for seniors and the disabled, and includes unwanted fondling, kissing, exhibitionism, harassment, and rape.

121. B: Terminals must be placed where others cannot read notes as they are typed. Much paperwork has been replaced by computerized charting, which is more legible, tamper-proof, and reduces errors by signaling if a treatment is missed or the wrong treatment is provided. Computer terminals often link to both patient databases and clinical decision support systems (CDSS), which provide diagnosis and treatment options based on the patient's symptoms. A point-of-care terminal is located at the patient's bedside. More terminals are placed at nursing stations, procedure rooms, and stock rooms. Easy access and comfortable height are ergonomically important, but remember that HIPAA requires *all* health facility staff protect confidential patient information. Situate computer terminals where passersby cannot read notes as you compose them. Computer access must be password protected and a timed-out screen saver must prevent unauthorized oversight when you leave the terminal temporarily.

122. A: Alginate. Brown seaweed is manufactured into wafers, sheets, fibers, and ropes for medical purposes. Alginate absorbs large amounts of wound drainage and forms a hydrophilic gel that conforms to the wound's shape. Alginate is effective for large wounds with undermining and tunneling, such as pressure ulcers. Hydrogel, which provides moisture, is used for dry and/or necrotic wounds, or those with minimal drainage. Hydrocolloid sheets and wafers provide an occlusive dressing for clean, granulated wounds with small to moderate amounts of drainage. Semi-permeable film is used primarily to protect skin under IVs or dry, shallow, partial thickness wounds, because it does not absorb drainage.

123. A: Puppet, doll, and needle play. During early childhood, children learn by participation, such as role-playing, simple explanation, and teaching dolls. Allowing children to play with medical equipment under supervision can allay some of their fears and help them to understand upcoming procedures. Needle play, in which the child gives "shots" to a doll with safe plastic syringes, can help him or her to express feelings about repeated blood draws or injections. When the NP provides dolls and puppets and engages in role play, it may encourage the worried child to express anxiety and fear through "talking" for the toy.

124. C: Prealbumin. Prealbumin is also called transthyretin. It has a half-life of only two or three days, so levels quickly decrease when nutrition is inadequate, and it reflects short-term protein deficiencies. Prealbumin levels rise quickly in response to increased protein intake. Albumin has a half-life of 18 to 20 days, so it is more sensitive as a marker of long-term protein deficiencies. Total protein levels can be influenced by many factors, including stress and infection, so total protein is monitored as part of an overall nutritional

assessment. Transferrin has a half-life of 8 to 10 days, but transferrin levels are sensitive to many different things, so levels are not always reliable indicators of nutritional status.

125. A: Methods to avoid gangs, tobacco, drugs, alcohol, and abusive relationships. Anticipatory guidance for early adolescence (11 to 14 years) should include helping the child go through socio-behavioral changes. Ask the child about social groups and pressures at school. Discuss methods to avoid gangs, tobacco, drugs, alcohol, and abusive relationships. Also outline what the child should expect in terms of bodily changes and development of secondary sexual characteristics (hair growth, acne, hormonally-induced mood swings, voice deepening, muscle and fat distribution, and sexual urges). Anticipatory guidance during older adolescence (15 to 17 years) includes discussing sexual responsibility (abstinence and birth control), relationships with family and peers, risk-taking behavior (smoking, drinking, drugs, and promiscuity), and future goals.

126. A: Female with a waist circumference of 37 inches. A female whose waist circumference exceeds 35 inches, or a male whose waist exceeds 40 inches, are at high risk for cardiovascular disease and diabetes. A person with a large waist tends to have increased risk even if his or her BMI is within normal limits. Although BMI is based on height and weight, it doesn't measure fat directly. A sedentary person may replace muscle with fat and still maintain a normal BMI. However, BMI provides a quick and easy estimate of the patient's health for the nurse practitioner. A BMI less than 18.5 indicates your patient is underweight. A BMI between 18.5 to 24.9 is within the normal range for both males and females. A BMI equal to or greater than 25 means your patient is overweight. If your patient has a BMI of 30, then he is obese. A patient with a BMI of 40 pr more is morbidly obese.

127. B: Nocturnal polysomnography. Book your patient at a sleep lab to assess him for obstructive sleep apnea syndrome (OSAS), which results from passive collapse of the pharynx during sleep. OSAS is often associated with a narrowed or restricted upper airway from micrognathia, obesity, or enlarged tonsils. It is most common in middle-aged, overweight males, and is exacerbated by ingesting alcohol or sedative drugs before sleeping. Signs and symptoms of OSAS include daytime somnolence, headache, cognitive impairment, depression, personality changes, recent increase in weight, and impotence. OSAS patients often snore loudly. They have cycles of breath cessation (apneic periods) up to 60 seconds long, occurring at least 30 times per night, despite continued chest wall and abdominal movements, indicating automatic attempts to breathe.

128. D: High-sensitivity FOBT annually, flexible sigmoidoscopy every 5 years, and colonoscopy every 10 years. Current guidelines for colorectal cancer screening include a high-sensitive FOBT annually, a flexible sigmoidoscopy every 5 years, and a colonoscopy every 10 years for *asymptomatic* patients between the ages of 50 and 75. Patients with symptoms, such as GI bleeding, require more frequent colonoscopies. High-risk patients, such as those with inflammatory bowel disease and alcoholism, need screening earlier and more frequently. Consider screening patients older than 75 on an individual basis, depending on their risk factors and health history. Most patients older than 80 have diverticula that make investigations more uncomfortable and dangerous.

129. A: Poverty. Poverty is probably the primary factor responsible for this mother delaying her child's medical care. She may not have personal health insurance and may not qualify for state medical assistance. Perhaps she is unaware that her daughter is eligible, so she may not take her child for care even if it is available. Most likely this homeless mother lacks

an automobile, or has insufficient funds for public transportation, or their shelter is inaccessible to public transportation. Since her mother has attempted to treat her child with over-the-counter meds, neglect does not seem to be the primary factor.

130. B: Creatinine clearance. A creatinine clearance test is indicated prior to an MRI with gadolinium because gadolinium is cleared through the kidneys. Gadolinium is a paramagnetic metal ion associated with nephrogenic systemic fibrosis in patients with impaired renal function. Gadolinium alters the magnetic field, producing different signals that translate into clearer images for the radiologist. While requirements for routine testing vary from one lab to another, most labs require testing of patients older than 60, especially for those who have a history of chronic illness. Stay alert for the chronic diseases that damage kidneys, such as diabetes, renal disease, and hypertension.

131. C: Respite care. *Respite care* relieves the stress of the family member who provides long-term care at home for a patient who is chronically or terminally ill. Hospice regulations allow the patient admission to a skilled nursing facility for up to five days, while the caregiver recovers. Some respite programs provide a nurse aide to stay with the patient for a few hours, while the caregiver leaves the home. Other respite programs provide money to the caregiver to independently hire part-time help in the home.

132. C: She must change to a birth control pill containing estrogen *and* use spermicide with her diaphragm. Isotretinoin is an effective acne medication, but it is also a powerful teratogen that causes serious birth defects. Its adverse effects on a developing fetus include mental retardation, facial malformation, hearing and vision defects. Isotretinoin interferes with progesterone-only birth control pills, so she is insufficiently protected from conception. Your patient must use acceptable primary *and* secondary forms of birth control in order to take isotretinoin safely. Dispense an estrogen-containing birth control pill *and* a spermicide foam or gel to her. Show her how to use the spermicide effectively with her diaphragm. Explain that she must use consistent birth control and have two negative pregnancy tests *prior* to starting treatment. Schedule her for a laboratory-based pregnancy test every month during treatment with isotretinoin *and* for one month after treatment stops.

133. A: Non-English speaking patient. The ability to speak English has nothing to do with taking medications as prescribed, since a competent translator can provide the necessary information. Directly-observed therapy (DOT) for TB is most often provided for:
- Positive sputum cultures for acid-fast bacilli
- Co-morbid conditions requiring concurrent treatment with antiretroviral (HIV) drugs or methadone (for heroin addiction)
- Multi-drug resistant (MDR) TB and extremely drug resistant (XDR) TB
- Co-morbid psychiatric disease that renders the patient unreliable for compliance
- Cognitive impairment
- Homelessness or lack of adequate facilities
- Demonstrated lack of reliability in taking treatments
- Twice weekly instead of daily administration

134. D: Abdominal ultrasound. Noninvasive abdominal ultrasound is most indicated, as her symptoms are consistent with cholecystitis, and ultrasound will show calculi. Her liver function tests may be within normal range, especially if she has no blockage of the common

bile duct. A cholangiogram may be used intraoperatively, especially if she has common bile duct blockage. An MRI is expensive, but may be necessary if the ultrasound is inconclusive. Cholecystitis with calculi can result in severe colic from obstruction of the bile duct, and pancreatitis from obstruction of the pancreatic duct. Cholecystitis is most common in overweight women between 20 and 40, and especially likely in those who are "fat, fair, and 40".

135. D: Cold packs on his neck, groin, and axillae. A patient suffering with heat exhaustion requires rehydration and mild cooling techniques, such as cold packs applied to the neck, groin, and axillae, or evaporative cooling by spraying him with cool water. You may also remove his clothes and wrap him in a wet sheet. Alcohol baths are no longer advised and are considered dangerous. Rapid cooling techniques, such as ice bath immersion and intravascular cooling, are only used if the patient has indications of heat stroke. Symptoms of heat stroke are similar, but extend to altered mental status, collapse, confusion and/or hallucinations, because of the CNS involvement.

136. D: Providing resolution. Some intermittent problems, such as cardiac arrhythmias, can improve with treatment, so the goals will aim toward resolution: "Pulse rate will not exceed 90 at rest." Maintaining status quo suggests taking no action at all to resolve a problem. Other problems that are chronic probably won't resolve, so the goals will aim toward preventing deterioration or further complications: "Patient will maintain current weight." Some problems, such as terminal cancer, cannot be resolved and deterioration of the patient's condition is inevitable. The goals will aim toward palliation and ensuring the end-stage patient's comfort and support: "Patient will not experience breakthrough pain."

137. D: Attending Alcoholics Anonymous. Primary prevention is taking steps before a disease occurs, such as by having immunizations and routine screening tests. Secondary prevention is taking steps after a disease occurs, or after risk factors are identified, to slow the progression of a disease. Secondary prevention may include: Modifying the diet and increasing exercise to reduce weight; taking Aspirin and antihypertensives to prevent another heart attack; or modifying work and activities to reduce stress. These prevention methods are not mutually exclusive, but may all be applied. Tertiary prevention is taking steps to manage chronic disorders, including attending support groups, such as Alcoholics Anonymous®, and rehabilitation programs.

138. B: Abdominal CT. Diverticulosis is a condition in which diverticula (sac-like outpouchings of the bowel lining that extend through a defect in the muscle layer) occur within the GI tract. Diverticulitis occurs as diverticula become inflamed when food or bacteria are retained within diverticula, resulting in abscess, obstruction from calculi, perforation, bleeding, or fistula. A CT scan confirms diverticulitis. A barium enema will show the presence of diverticular outpouchings, but not inflammation. A stool specimen may show the presence of occult blood, but the results are non-specific. Leucocytosis is present with diverticulitis but is also non-specific.

139. A: Tics must be present for four weeks but no longer than one year. Transient tick disorder is very common, affecting almost 25% of children. Transient tics are present for at least four weeks but no longer than one year. Chronic tic disorder persists longer than one year. Movement tics (blinking, jerking, grimacing, and sticking the tongue out) are more common than vocal tics (grunting, sniffing, clearing throat, and squealing). Tic behavior is more common during the winter months (November through February), although the

reason is unclear. Tics are generally absent during sleep in transient tic disorder, but are evident in all stages of sleep with chronic tic disorder.

140. D: The patient is eligible for Medicare A, and a physician certifies the patient has a life expectancy of six months or less. In order to obtain hospice (end-of-life) care, the Medicare patient must be eligible for Medicare A, *and* a physician must certify him as terminal. The initial prognosis must be a life expectancy of less than 6 months, although this may be extended by the physician's authorization every 60 days. Medicare requires the patient to agree to receive palliative hospice care, rather than regular curative treatment. The goal of hospice care is to maintain the patient comfortably in his own home environment. Therefore, the patient is provided with: Home health aides for personal care; homemakers for cleaning, shopping, and laundry; durable goods (dressings, adult diapers, and under pads); pain management; case management; psychological counseling; and Social Work assistance. Routine home care is intermittent and must comprise 80% of the patient's total care.

141. B: Use an expressive vocabulary of four to six words, but understand many more words, and point to something desired, such as a toy. A 12-month old is still largely nonverbal, but should be able to say a few words with comprehension, such as "Mama," and "Dada," and imitate some animal sounds. A 13 to 15-month old child increases to a four to six word expressive vocabulary, and understands many more words. By 13 to 15 months, the toddler should point to indicate a desire for something, such as a toy. A 16 to 18-month old should be able to use a 7 to 20-word vocabulary and point to five body parts. A 20-month old should combine two words, and is more verbal, with about half of his vocabulary understandable by the caregiver. A 24-month old should understand 300 words and use sentences of two or three words in length.

142. A: Rosenberg's non-violent communication. OFNR follows Rosenberg's non-violent communication (NVC) model. OFNR means observing without making judgments, expressing feelings about observations, expressing needs associated with feelings, and making requests to meet needs. The continuous loop model includes content and a sender who uses the content to send a message to a receiver, who then provides feedback to the sender. The Shannon and Weaver communication model includes the sender as the information source, transmitter as means of communication, noise (mental or other interference) and a receiver, who may receive an altered or confused message. Berlo's communication process includes the source, encoder (sound producer), message, channel (message medium), decoder (translating skills), and receiver.

143. A: "I have a cataract growing on the outside of my eye." Cataracts do not grow *on* the eye. Therefore, the patient needs education to understand that only the lens of the affected eye is becoming cloudy or opaque, and the lack of clarity interferes with vision. The National Eye Institute's Age-Related Eye Disease Study confirmed that multivitamin supplements that include zinc, copper, Vitamin C, Vitamin E, and Vitamin A (AREDS formula) reduce the incidence of age-related macular degeneration. Warm compresses (4 to 6 times daily for 15 minutes each) are standard treatment for styes. Disposable contact lenses are changed either daily or every two weeks, depending on the brand.

144. A: Contact Child Protective Services within 24 hours. Nurse Practitioners are mandated reporters. You are required by law to notify Child Protective Services of your suspicions, so the proper authorities can investigate the possibility of child abuse. Spiral fractures of the

shafts of long bones are the most common abuse-related fracture in children. Additionally, new bruises should be red-purple. Widespread yellow-green and brown bruises suggest earlier injuries. A three-year-old child is not a reliable reporter. Do not forewarn the mother by questioning her about abuse. Giving advice may cause an abusive mother to remove the child from care to avoid detection.

145. D: Standard audiometry. Standard audiometry with earphones that emit sounds is usually appropriate for children older than 5 years and adults. Auditory brainstem response (ABR), which uses scalp electrodes to measure the brain's reaction to sound, is used for infants. Another test for infants is otoacoustic emissions (OAE), which uses a probe in the ear to measure sounds generated by the cochlea. Visual reinforcement audiometry (VRA) rewards a child 6 to 24 months old with a moving toy or light, when the child looks toward a sound. Conditioned play audiometry (CPA) requires the toddler (2 to 5 years old) to watch a demonstration and then do a particular activity when hearing a sound.

146. D: A lactose-free diet. A lactose-free diet helps patients with GI symptoms from lactose intolerance. A lactose-free diet does not help to prevent heart disease or rehabilitate those with existing heart disease. The goal of secondary prevention is to improve the patient's quality of life, increase the survival rate, reduce the need for procedures, and decrease the incidence of heart attack. Secondary prevention strategies include an exercise program, diabetic management, smoking cessation, lipid management, weight control, and medications to control hypertension and prevent blood clots, including ASA, ARBS, ACEIs, ⍰-blockers, and antiplatelet agents.

147. C: Lumbar puncture and examination of his cerebrospinal fluid. Your patient's symptoms are consistent with bacterial meningitis. The correct diagnostic test for meningitis is a lumbar puncture and examination of cerebrospinal fluid. Kernig's and Brudzinski's signs are specific to meningitis and rarely occur with other disorders:
- Kernig's sign: Flex the patient's hips. Then, try to straighten the knees while the hips are flexed. Hamstring spasms make this painful and difficult for a patient with meningitis.
- Brudzinski's sign: Position the child lying supine. Flex the child's neck by pulling the head toward the chest. Neck stiffness (nuchal rigidity) causes the hips and knees to pull up into a flexed position if the patient has meningitis.

148. A: Roll over, roll from back to side, turn his head from any position, and sit with support for 10 to 15 minutes. At 6 months, an infant should be able to: Roll over; roll from back to side; hold his head up at a 90⍰⍰angle; turn his head in both directions when lying and sitting; and sit with support for 10 to 15 minutes. Expected mobility at other ages is as follows:
- 4 months: Lift head while prone or supine; turn head from side to side; and roll stomach to back
- 8 months: Sit alone; stand while supported, and bounce on legs
- 10 moths: Crawl or creep readily; sit up; and pull up to standing position

149. D: Accept resistance to change. Motivational interviewing (MI) techniques include accepting resistance to change as normal, suggesting the counselor needs to modify his or her approaches. MI focuses on motivation for change originating from the client. An MI counselor avoids trying to persuade or confront the client to change unwanted behaviors. MI considers the therapeutic relationship a partnership, in which the counselor avoids the

role of expert. The counselor helps the client identify ambivalence (such as the life desired, as opposed to the life lived), but leaves resolution up to the client.

150. A: The entire population. According to the WHO principles of health promotion, activities should focus on the entire population as they normally live their lives, rather than a specific high-risk group. WHO recommends looking at the determinants and causes of disease, and applying diverse methods and approaches to promote health. Health promotion should focus on social and political efforts to engage the public in participation, rather than to provide medical service. For example, widely successful health promotion activities include smoking cessation and seat belt use.

Practice Test #2

Practice Questions

1. The nurse practitioner is educating an adult patient regarding medications for asthma. Which order would be the most appropriate for administration?
   a. Flovent, Intal, Tobramycin
   b. Tobramycin, Intal, Albuterol
   c. Albuterol, Flovent, Tobramycin
   d. Intal, Tobramycin, Albuterol

2. What are the best question types to ask when gaining information from a patient?
   a. specific, open-ended questions regarding current symptoms and medical history
   b. general questions with yes or no answers
   c. questions related to childhood diseases
   d. demographics questions

3. In what order would you prioritize the care of the following patients presenting to your office at the same time: a parent carrying a smiling infant with a fever, a pale and sweaty male with flank pain for two days, a carpenter with a nail in his thumb, and a three-year-old with vomiting.
   a. flank pain, infant with fever, three-year-old with vomiting, and man with the nail
   b. flank pain, three-year-old with vomiting, infant with a fever, and man with the nail
   c. three-year-old with vomiting, infant with fever, flank pain, and man with the nail
   d. three-year-old with vomiting, flank pain, man with the nail, and infant with fever

4. Mom has described her child's symptoms as fever for three days and vomiting for the last 24 hours. She states the child has been very sleepy for the last two to three hours. What subtle symptom alerts the nurse practitioner that this child needs to be seen as soon as possible?
   a. three days of fever
   b. three days of fever, one day of vomiting
   c. one day of vomiting,
   d. very sleepy for two to three hours with a fever for three days

5. A nurse practitioner takes a phone call from the daughter of a 60-year-old male stating that he isn't himself today. When questioned further, the nurse practitioner discovers that the man has had periods of slurred speech for a few minutes on two occasions in the last 24 hours. What is your recommendation for this caller regarding what should be done for her father?
   a. You understand that slurred speech may be the result of too much alcohol or lack of sleep, and you encourage her to call back again if it reoccurs.
   b. You advise her to come in to the office in the next 24–48 hours for some blood work.
   c. You advise her that slurred speech may be a symptom of a transient ischemic attack (TIA) or impending stroke, especially in relation to his "not being himself" and to go to the nearest emergency room.
   d. You tell her you will call her back when you can consult with a physician.

6. A 70-year-old female presents to the office complaining of fatigue. You begin your assessment, and she has a heart rate of 50, a respiratory rate of 24, and a blood pressure of 70/40. She denies chest pain, but you notice she rubs her elbows and states her arthritis is acting up. What would be your first priority when caring for this patient?
   a. Offer her Tylenol for pain and send her to the waiting room.
   b. Offer her Motrin for pain.
   c. Continue her assessment and history and finish the paperwork.
   d. Place her in a room, do an electrocardiogram (EKG), and place her before the other patients in the office because of the possibility of a heart problem.

7. What nonverbal clues would indicate that a patient of any age is having difficulty breathing?
   a. change in color, retractions, and noisy breathing
   b. laughing and joking during a triage assessment
   c. slight wheezing when lifting heavy objects
   d. sweating in a warm room with exertion

8. What would be the most appropriate order of importance for information an adult client shares when coming to a office visit?
   a. past medical history, past surgical history, medications, allergies, and insurance information
   b. current complaint, past 24–48 hours leading up to complaint, medications, allergies, and past medical history
   c. current medications, allergies, past medical history, and past surgical history
   d. current demographics, current insurance, complaint, medical history, and surgical history

9. A 50-year-old male comes to the office stating he cannot shake this "flu." You observe that he is clammy, pale, and has an irregular heart rate. He is a large man with a rugged appearance. He is friendly and apologetic for bothering you with his silly complaints. What is your plan of care for this patient?
   a. You suspect he has a low tolerance for being ill and offer him Tylenol while he waits.
   b. You suspect he has the newest flu going around and offer him hot tea while he waits.
   c. You suspect there is more to his complaint than he states and immediately begin a cardiac workup.
   d. You finish the assessment understanding that the flu affects everyone differently.

10. What is the most appropriate way to ask a patient about possible physical abuse during the triage process?
   a. Ask questions regarding abuse in front of the spouse, so there is a witness.
   b. Never ask if the information is not offered; it is an invasion of privacy.
   c. Ask the patient directly without the spouse or parent in the room.
   d. Begin by describing your own experience in an attempt to get the patient to open up.

11. A mother bringing her teenager into the office is concerned that the child has a fruity odor to her breath and is sleepy more than usual. The child seems to skip meals and become nauseated frequently. What on-site, quick laboratory test may give an initial idea about what might be causing the fruity breath and sleepiness?
   a. urine dipstick
   b. urine dipstick and glucometer
   c. glucometer
   d. rapid strep test

12. What would be the most valid reason for performing a streptococcal throat culture in the office setting for a patient with a fever and sore throat?
   a. To protect the liability of the clinicians in the facility.
   b. To provide protection for the staff from clients who may carry strep.
   c. It is a low-cost way to diagnose and get antibiotics initiated quickly.
   d. It is a billable service and can bring in revenue to the clinic.

13. An adult male presents to the office setting with a 24-hour history of wheezing, coughing, and shortness of breath. What would be the most appropriate invasive procedure that he may require from the nurse in this setting?
   a. blood glucose monitoring
   b. urine dipstick
   c. blood pressure monitoring
   d. a nebulizer treatment

14. Which noninvasive procedure is part of a routine school physical for students in kindergarten that can be performed in an office setting?
   a. vision exam
   b. immunizations
   c. strep test
   d. occult blood test

15. An 18-year-old female presents to the office complaining of pelvic pain and foul discharge. What would be the most appropriate nursing interventions for this patient?
   a. The woman may not be treated at an outpatient office because she is a minor.
   b. The nurse understands that the patient should be referred to a gynecologist, and the nurse can refuse to treat the patient.
   c. The nurse practitioner will refer the patient to Planned Parenthood or another free clinic in her area rather than evaluate her.
   d. The nurse practitioner protects the privacy of the female by taking her to a private room doing a complete assessment and history, and prepares the patient for a pelvic exam.

16. What best describes the advantages of doing on-site testing for patients, such as glucose monitoring, urine tests, rapid strep cultures, or blood tests to diagnose flulike symptoms?
    a. Early diagnosis and prevention are cost-effective for the client, the facility, and the insurance providers.
    b. It gives the facility extra means to bring in cash by testing all patients for common disorders.
    c. There is no financial advantage, but it is convenient for the patient.
    d. The testing should not be done in an office setting because the outcomes are not accurate.

17. What would be the result of improper sterilization or disinfection of equipment in the office setting?
    a. no result that could be identified
    b. the transfer of bacteria to another patient or staff member
    c. room air will destroy most bacteria after 48 hours
    d. not enough data are available to infer a reasonable answer

18. A parent brings her teenage son into the office stating that he has been wheezing for a day or two with no history of asthma. The boy does not appear to be in distress but does have an audible wheeze. What noninvasive procedure might a nurse practitioner consider as part of the physical assessment?
    a. chest X-ray
    b. a peak flow meter reading
    c. a blood glucose level
    d. a urinalysis for drug screening

19. The nurse practitioner is caring for a young mother and her toddler. Which statement demonstrates that primary prevention is part of the role of the nurse practitioner?
    a. The practitioner discusses seat belt safety with the mother and offers to show her the proper use of car seat restraints.
    b. The practitioner offers the mother a magazine and a drink while she waits to be evaluated.
    c. The practitioner performs the assessment on both the mother and the child.
    d. The practitioner documents the current immunization status of the child.

20. A nurse practitioner working in the office is offering patient education to a 50-year-old male client. Which statement demonstrates an understanding of the meaning of secondary prevention?
    a. The nurse practitioner asks the patient to return again when and if his pain reoccurs.
    b. The nurse practitioner explains the importance of early diagnosis and treatment for colon cancer and encourages him to make an appointment for a colonoscopy.
    c. The nurse practitioner performs her assessment and proceeds to discuss his lab results.
    d. Secondary prevention is not related to ambulatory care and is not discussed by the nurse practitioner in the office setting.

21. What disease entity/client would respond best with a consistent continuity of care over a longer length of time?
    a. a new mom with a healthy newborn
    b. an elderly diabetic who lives with her daughter
    c. a noncompliant teen with sickle cell anemia whose single-parent mom works
    d. a toddler with chicken pox

22. Which statement correctly demonstrates the responsibility of the nurse practitioner to a chronically ill patient?
    a. The nurse practitioner has little responsibility when it comes to the chronically ill.
    b. The nurse practitioner realizes that wellness education is still an important part of treating the client who has a chronic illness and includes that in her plan of care.
    c. The nurse practitioner will refer any chronically ill client because there are no treatments to implement that would enhance recovery.
    d. The nurse practitioner realizes that the cost of care is decreased when a patient is chronically ill.

23. Which statement demonstrates the nurse practitioner using outside resources when providing client care?
    a. The nurse practitioner refers the client to a government-funded program that will provide food for his or her infant.
    b. The nurse practitioner recommends checking the Internet for further education and information.
    c. Statements a and b both show utilization of outside resources.
    d. The nurse practitioner does not refer the client to outside resources, preferring to offer all treatment and education at office.

24. Which statement best describes understanding the role of nurse practioner in the cost of care for clients?
    a. The nurse practitioner needs a degree in accounting before being part of the financial committee.
    b. The cost of care is not the responsibility of the nurse practitioner.
    c. The nurse practitioner understands that reimbursement for some interventions may differ in acute illness versus when the patient is well, and that prevention can be cost-effective.
    d. Case management is very expensive and is reserved for the acute care setting.

25. A nurse practitioner refers a client to the community hospital education program for new diabetics. Which category of care management does this fall under?
    a. treatment
    b. implementation
    c. coordination
    d. utilization of resources

26. The nurse practitioner practicing in office setting understands that performance improvement becomes part of the responsibility of the health-care team. Which item would be a performance improvement indicator for an office and the health-care team?
   a. payroll
   b. critical pathways
   c. marketing brochures
   d. staff schedules

27. The nurse practitioner is treating a female patient for symptoms of fever and body aches. The patient also has cancer. What statement describes the practitioner's role in collaboration with other members of the health-care team—including oncology?
   a. The nurse practitioner must document the symptoms and has no obligation to relate the information to another facility.
   b. The nurse practitioner will make sure the office is aware that the client is also an oncology patient.
   c. The nurse practitioner understands that collaboration means working toward a common goal, in this case, the care of an oncology client. Sharing knowledge about the symptoms would include consulting with the client's oncologist to help resolve the problem and deciding on a diagnosis and treatment plan specific to this patient.
   d. Past medical history or current relationships to other medical specialties are not related to giving care at an office location.

28. Which statement would describe the use of the Internet as a resource for an nurse practitioner or patient?
   a. a source of educational information
   b. a distraction for when the patient load is light
   c. a way to order meals when the staff is too busy
   d. The Internet is not used in the ambulatory care setting for information.

29. What resources that may be offered by the nurse practitioner as a part of the treatment plan would be helpful to a client presenting with a domestic abuse problem?
   a. scheduling a return appointment at the office
   b. community resources including churches, women's shelters, and legal aid
   c. job or work programs
   d. the police department

30. The nurse practitioner is taking care of a pediatric patient who presents with general complaints. During the course of the initial treatment, the child appears to be getting sicker. What would be the action for the nurse practitioner caring for this client?
   a. The nurse practitioner would continue to care for all the patients in order of presenting to the clinic.
   b. The nurse practitioner would assign someone to reassess the child frequently.
   c. The nurse practitioner would assess the child and be ready to transfer him or her to a primary or specialty facility that handles emergency care.
   d. The nurse practitioner would instruct the parent to return to the facility if the child's symptoms get worse.

31. A young adult male presents to the office complaining of blood in his urine after working out at the gym. Which statement regarding blood in the urine should the nurse practitioner consider when managing the treatment plan and implementation for this client and advocating for his care?
   a. Occasional blood in the urine can be overlooked and requires no treatment.
   b. Blood in the urine can be an indication of muscle breakdown and can represent kidney damage. Treatment and follow-up care should be considered.
   c. Blood in the urine always indicates infection and requires antibiotic therapy.
   d. Male clients do not have blood in their urine.

32. A female client presents to the clinic with shortness of breath for the past six months. She states that she smokes one pack of cigarettes a day. Which statement best describes the patient advocacy role the nurse practitioner would assume in this situation?
   a. providing patient education
   b. providing mechanisms to measure patient satisfaction
   c. providing access to care
   d. providing continuity of care

33. A client presents to the facility despondent and having suicidal thoughts. What role does the nurse practitioner have in treating this client?
   a. The nurse practitioner has no special role.
   b. The nurse practitioner should help to assure that the client has the right access, right provider, the right time frame for treatment, and the right level of care for the symptoms and complaint presented.
   c. The nurse practitioner should make certain the client received a patient satisfaction survey upon leaving.
   d. The nurse practitioner should ensure that security is on site, due to the mental state of the client.

34. The nurse practitioner understands that patient satisfaction is subjective. What measurement indicator will assist in evaluating the data collected?
   a. Making certain that there is a complaint resolution process in place and an atmosphere of objectivity and specific ways to deal with the data allow for improvement in the future.
   b. The nurse practitioner has little to do with the collection of data or the results of the data.
   c. The nurse practitioner does not use measurement indicators to determine if a patient is happy with the care; rather, he or she bases satisfaction on the end result of the diagnosis.
   d. The nurse practitioner measures the number of good outcomes against the bad outcomes and then gets the percent of satisfied clients from that data.

35. The nurse practitioner is caring for clients of different ages, abilities, and levels of health. Which skills would best help to be an effective advocate for the clients?
   a. being organized and able to multitask
   b. being able to telephone triage
   c. being cognitive about the fiscal status of the ambulatory facility
   d. being able to partner with the client, family, and the entire health-care team to provide the care needed for each age and disease state

36. The nurse practitioner explains the plan and obtains consents from the client before proceeding. Included in her discussion may be options for care. Which term best describes what the nurse's intentions are for the client?
    a. providing enough information so the client can make an informed decision
    b. to stall for time as he or she silently assesses the client
    c. to legally cover the basics to prevent a lawsuit later
    d. The practitioner is following the facility's policy.

37. The practitioner detects nonverbal signs of fear and distrust when triaging a female client in the presence of her male companion. What might she suspect is happening when the nonverbal behaviors of the female client are considered?
    a. The practitioner suspects the patient is anxious about being at the clinic and distrusts doctors.
    b. The practitioner suspects the injuries may not have occurred the way the client describes and should suspect domestic violence.
    c. The practitioner should not pay attention to nonverbal behavior and react only to what is being said.
    d. The practitioner suspects nothing.

38. When the nurse practitioner suspects that domestic violence may be the cause of injury, what is the best approach to communicating with the client to get an honest answer and to offer assistance?
    a. Continue asking appropriate questions about the injuries in front of the client's companion.
    b. Point-blank accuse the client of not being honest in an effort to make her confess.
    c. Take the client to a private exam area to continue questioning and offer assistance away from her companion.
    d. The nurse practitioner should report the suspected abuse without further probing.

39. The nurse practitioner understands which principle of communication when dealing with employees and peers?
    a. It is important to understand the various types of approaches used to manage conflict.
    b. Conflict should be dealt with honestly and openly with all team members.
    c. Understand that conflict resolution is an ongoing process within an interdisciplinary team an office care setting.
    d. All of the above statements are true.

40. The nurse practitioner shows cultural competence by which of the following actions?
    a. disregarding the desire for modesty shown by the females of some cultures by asking them to disrobe
    b. identifying and avoiding gestures that groups or cultures may find offensive
    c. failing to modify communication patterns to the style of the group addressed
    d. failing to use clarifying techniques when educating clients of another culture

41. The nurse practitioner showing cultural competency recognizes which statement to be true about the term "space" when interacting with clients of a different culture?
   a. Space means the outer atmosphere.
   b. Space differences are the same for all cultures.
   c. Space refers to distinct zones in relation to personal, intimate, and public space and has different meanings in different cultures.
   d. Space is irrelevant when dealing with a client who is ill and seeking medical care.

42. The nurse practitioner takes care of different ethnic groups of people under stress in a variety of situations in the clinic. What other factors influence the way the client reacts to the health-care team besides cultural background?
   a. socioeconomic background and level of education
   b. the number of family members accompanying the client
   c. the day of the week
   d. the visual appearance of the clinic

43. What would be a key aspect for the practitioner when caring for a variety of clients from different backgrounds?
   a. keeping quiet and ignoring the differences
   b. respecting each client
   c. getting a translator
   d. avoiding those you are not comfortable with

44. The nurse practitioner is giving instructions for medication and dressing changes to a Spanish-speaking client. What would be the most effective way to make certain the client understands the instructions?
   a. The nurse practitioner should have the client give a return demonstration.
   b. The nurse practitioner should use hand gestures to explain the procedure.
   c. The nurse practitioner should have a Spanish-speaking translator present when giving the instructions.
   d. The nurse practitioner should give instructions to the family as well as the client.

45. The client comes into the office and asks the nurse practitioner about a change in medication because the cost is too high. What could the nurse practitioner offer the client besides a different medication?
   a. The nurse practitioner may offer to pay for the prescription.
   b. The nurse practitioner may refer the client to community resources with addresses and phone numbers for agencies that may offer financial assistance.
   c. The nurse practitioner may suggest ways to prioritize the client's budget.
   d. The nurse practitioner does not usually get involved with payment issues, as it crosses the nurse/patient boundary.

46. The nurse practitioner must arrange a transfer for a male patient with chest pain. What are the appropriate actions the nurse practitioner must take to get the patient safely transferred?
   a. The nurse practitioner must call the acute care facility and give a report before the transfer can occur.
   b. The nurse practitioner gives the documentation to the doctor, and her job is done.
   c. The nurse practitioner communicates to other team members that a transfer will occur and goes to lunch.
   d. The nurse practitioner is not responsible for arranging the transfer; the responsibility falls to other team members.

47. The nurse practitioner uses a fax machine to gain information about a client from another facility. What must be included with the fax in order to obtain this information?
   a. a fax cover sheet
   b. a fax cover sheet and a signed release of information from the client
   c. a signed release of information
   d. There is no need for anything but a phone call to the facility.

48. What types of documentation would be appropriate for telephone encounters with a client or facility?
   a. telephone log, spiral notebook, or a note in the client chart
   b. Telephone encounters do not need documentation if the nurse is following a facility's protocol.
   c. both a and b
   d. neither a nor b

49. Documentation is an important part of the care of the patient or client. Which statements describe appropriate strategies for documentation?
1. Documentation shows the care given from all health-care providers involved.
2. Documentation should be as little as possible for legal reasons.
3. Documentation facilitates reimbursement.
4. Documentation provides a narrative record of a health episode and provides continuity of care.
   a. 1, 2, 3
   b. 1, 3, 4
   c. 3, 4,
   d. 2, 3, 4

50. The nurse practitioner understands that professional boundaries are part of the responsibility when relating to patients and families. Which statement demonstrates an understanding of those professional boundaries when a client asks the nurse practitioner about another client's diagnosis?
   a. The nurse practitioner ignores the question and continues doing something else.
   b. The nurse practitioner politely states that she is not allowed to discuss other clients for the protection of the client's privacy.
   c. The nurse practitioner may describe the diagnosis in generic terms, as long as he or she is not specific.
   d. The nurse practitioner may relay information if one client knows the other client outside of the clinic.

51. A woman makes an appointment with the clinic to discuss resources available to care for her elderly mother, who has suffered several strokes and has terminal cancer. What would be an appropriate consultation or referral source be for this client?
- a. social services
- b. oncologist
- c. hospice
- d. speech therapist

52. A teen complains of suicidal thoughts to the nurse practitioner. What would be the best action, within professional boundaries, that the nurse practitioner should take?
- a. The nurse practitioner would follow the facility's policy about referrals to behavioral medicine and notify parents or caregivers as well as document the client's complaints and plan.
- b. The nurse practitioner would notify the police immediately.
- c. The nurse practitioner would document the information and leave it up to the physician to decide.
- d. The nurse practitioner would discuss the client's complaints before deciding what to do.

53. Which behavioral management techniques for urinary incontinence may be within the professional boundaries of the nurse practitioner?
- a. prescribing medications
- b. referrals to surgeons
- c. ordering diagnostic testing
- d. education regarding pelvic muscle strengthening exercises and monitoring fluid intake

54. Which item does not show examples of leadership?
- a. promoting a professional standard of care
- b. being an example or role model for new nurse practitioners in the field
- c. encouraging team members to participate in shared governance
- d. refusing to acknowledge the importance of certification

55. What regulatory organization sets the standards and enforces rules regarding occupational safety and health?
- a. the health department
- b. the materials data board
- c. OSHA
- d. EEOC

56. Which government agency regulates H1N1, flu, HIV, and other diseases by written guidelines for a standard of care?
- a. ADA
- b. AHA
- c. CDC
- d. OSHA

57. Which statement is true regarding patient safety?
    a. Patient falls are a concern only in an acute care setting.
    b. Patient confidentiality is part of patient safety.
    c. Side effects of medication are part of patient education and have nothing to do with safety.
    d. There are no regulations on patient safety.

58. What is the benefit of the Health Care Financing Administration Common Procedure coding system?
    a. It creates jobs.
    b. It does not allow for consistent classification.
    c. It provides a method for health-care providers to be consistent and communicate services that have been rendered, so all get reimbursed equally for the same care.
    d. It does not allow for error.

59. What is the internationally recognized coding system for the purposes of international morbidity and mortality? In the United States, it is also used for billing.
    a. ICDSS
    b. ICD46
    c. ICDID
    d. ICD 9

60. What are examples of health-care delivery systems in terms of financial reimbursement?
    a. Fee for service is the only system.
    b. health maintenance organizations (HMOs), preferred provider organizations (PPOs), fee for service, and managed care
    c. Medicaid is the only system.
    d. Private insurance is the only system.

61. What is the most critical endpoint in a quality model in the delivery of health care?
    a. The patient is cured.
    b. The patient files no complaints.
    c. The care delivered made a difference in the outcome for the patient.
    d. Performance improvement cannot be measured.

62. What methods may improve performance and outcomes for a patient in the short or long term?
    a. evidence-based practice
    b. national health initiatives, such as smoking prevention or weight management
    c. clinical pathways and protocols
    d. all of the above

63. The nurse practitioner is caring for a 12-year-old boy who weighs 185 pounds. What patient education may be included in the care of this child?
    a. diet and nutrition
    b. exercise and weight management
    c. both a and b, regardless of complaint
    d. neither a nor b, regardless of complaint

64. What learning principles should the nurse practitioner keep in mind when doing health education for a teenager?
    a.   Information must be age appropriate and geared toward the needs of the patient.
    b.   Education can be graphic to scare the teen into being compliant.
    c.   Education does not have to be culturally sensitive as long as it is factual.
    d.   Education can be in the form of only reading material to save time.

65. The nurse practitioner is giving a community education program on smoking. What factors will determine how to present the information?
    a.   the age of the participants
    b.   the educational level of the participants
    c.   the socioeconomic status of the audience
    d.   all of the above

66. The nurse practitioner is providing education on teenage pregnancy to a group of older teens. What would be the appropriate principles to consider when discussing this subject?
    a.   the grade level of the group
    b.   the mental development of the group
    c.   the information requested by parents and teachers
    d.   all of the above

67. The nurse practitioner is discussing obesity and heart disease with a 50-year-old female. What information should the nurse practitioner include in the patient education?
    a.   Diet, exercise, and the relationship of obesity to heart disease.
    b.   Diets high in carbohydrates are best, especially if you don't exercise.
    c.   Exercise is not safe over the age of 50.
    d.   Chest pain is common in this age group.

68. The nurse practitioner is instructing the patient on the use of inhalers for her asthma. What should the nurse include in the patient education?
    a.   Teach the patient that asthma is not a serious illness.
    b.   Asthma can be managed, but compliance is essential.
    c.   There is no order in which inhalers should be taken.
    d.   Thrush is common, and there is no way to prevent it.

69. Emesis is a common occurrence in newborns. What condition should be considered if a 6 week old male infant presents with refractory, projectile emesis?
    a.   GE reflux
    b.   Pyloric stenosis
    c.   Appendicitis
    d.   Pancreatitis

70. A patient with acute infectious diarrhea has a fever and blood in his stool. His condition does not improve with oral hydration therapy. Which of the following is a risk factor for infection with *Clostridium difficile*?
    a.   Recent travel outside the U.S.
    b.   History of liver transplant
    c.   Daycare attendance
    d.   Use of antibiotics in the past six weeks

71. In elderly patients with complaints of constipation who have no other gastrointestinal abnormalities, the initial treatment should include all of the following *except*:
   a. Stimulant laxative
   b. Increased exercise
   c. Increased fiber intake from food sources
   d. Increased water intake

72. What would the best treatment be for a pre-partum woman at 36 weeks gestation that has a sprained ankle? Which of the following is NOT appropriate for pregnant women in the third trimester?
   a. Tylenol pm
   b. NSAID such as Ibuprofen or Naprosyn
   c. Ice
   d. Elevation

73. An eight year old female contracts chicken pox (varicella virus). Which of the following family members should she absolutely avoid to prevent their contracting the virus?
   a. Her two-year old brother who has had the varicella vaccine
   b. Her ninety year old great-grandmother
   c. Her twenty-year old uncle on chemotherapy
   d. Her twin sister

74. Which statement by a client identifies a need for further education after evaluating the client's cholesterol panel?
   a. "I need to raise my LDL level"
   b. "I need to raise my HDL level"
   c. "I need to lower my triglyceride level"
   d. "My ALT level needs to be lower"

75. A client is leaving on a long transatlantic flight. Which activities should the nurse advise the client to avoid?
   a. Staying well hydrated
   b. Walking intermittently in the aisles
   c. Wearing loose clothing
   d. Staying as still as possible

76. While counseling a mother of a one year old at a clinic visit, which statement indicates the need for further education?
   a. "Candy should be limited"
   b. "Sugared sodas should be avoided"
   c. "Apple juice in the nighttime bottle is acceptable"
   d. "I should check and see if our water is fluorinated"

77. A nurse practitioner is counseling the mother of a one year old client. The household is bilingual and the two languages are spoken equally to the child. What should the nurse practitioner advise regarding the development of speech in the child compared to children in households where the relatives speak only one language?
   a. The child's speech will likely start earlier
   b. The child's speech may start later
   c. There is no difference
   d. The child may not speak both languages as an adult

78. A nurse practitioner counsels a client with a UTI regarding OTC means of helping the condition in addition to the antibiotics prescribed. Which is NOT an appropriate intervention?
   a. Phenazopyridine (Pyridium)
   b. Cranberry extract pills
   c. Carbonated sodas
   d. Cranberry juice

79. As part of counseling for a child with mild persistent asthma, the nurse practitioner tells the client's family that the most reliable indicator of worsening asthma is:
   a. Sneezing
   b. Fever
   c. Decreased peak flow
   d. Pedal edema

80. Which of the following acne treatments requires female clients to use 2 forms of contraception and sign a consent form?
   a. Benzoyl peroxide cream
   b. Tetracycline (Sumycin) pills
   c. Isotretinoin (Accutane) pills
   d. Laser treatment

81. In order to swab a client's throat for a culture; the nurse practitioner can have the client do what to help prevent gagging?
   a. Hold open eyelids with fingers
   b. Hold nose
   c. Pull backwards on ears
   d. Hold breath

82. In order to collect proper blood culture samples, the nurse practitioner should do which of the following?
   a. Sterilize antecubital fossa with Iodine
   b. Draw sample from femoral site
   c. Wipe culture bottles with alcohol pad
   d. Shave collection site

83. As part of a pre-placement exam for employment, a client gets a PPD (Mantoux) skin test. When should the client return for reading of the result?
   a.   12 to 24 hours
   b.   24 to 48 hours
   c.   48 to 72 hours
   d.   72 to 96 hours

84. An elderly client with a skin tear on the forearm has a Tegaderm bandage placed on the area. What does the nurse practitioner tell the client regarding changing the bandage?
   a.   Change it every 8 hours
   b.   Wash the bandaged area bid
   c.   Leave the bandage on until seen by the physician
   d.   Wrap a tight Kerlix bandage on the area

85. A client with a history of GERD asks about non-pharmacological methods of helping his condition. Which of the following is NOT an appropriate intervention?
   a.   Decreasing caffeine
   b.   Increasing carbonated beverages
   c.   Decreasing alcohol
   d.   Losing weight

86. A client is taking several medications for different medical problems. Which of the following would NOT require periodic monitoring for blood levels?
   a.   Furosemide (Lasix)
   b.   Digoxin (Lanoxin)
   c.   Lithium (Lithobid)
   d.   Warfarin (Coumadin)

87. A pregnant client is advised to increase the amount of iron in her diet due to mild anemia. All of the following foods are high in iron *except* for:
   a.   Spinach
   b.   Beef
   c.   Rice
   d.   Lamb

88. A nurse practitioner is counseling teenage females about ways to prevent contracting human papilloma virus (HPV). All of the following are acceptable ways to decrease the spread of HPV *except*:
   a.   IUDs
   b.   Condoms
   c.   Abstinence
   d.   Gardasil vaccine

89. A 35 year old female who has smoked one pack of cigarettes a day for the past 20 years comes into a clinic for contraceptive counseling. Which would be a poor choice for this patient?
   a.   Oral contraceptive pills
   b.   Condoms
   c.   Diaphragm
   d.   Contraceptive sponge

90. Which statement by a teenager on a clinic visit indicates the need for further evaluation and possible intervention?
   a. "I use laxatives to keep my weight down"
   b. "I get very moody during my menstrual periods"
   c. "I often get in arguments with my mother"
   d. "I find it hard to get up in the morning for school"

91. After the divorce of his parents a four year old starts to suck his thumb again. What psychological defense mechanism is the child using?
   a. Repression
   b. Rationalization
   c. Regression
   d. Transference

92. What newborn condition increases the risk of future testicular cancer if not corrected?
   a. Inguinal hernia
   b. Umbilical hernia
   c. Hirschsprung's megacolon
   d. Undescended testes

93. A mother brings in a teenage client, who is an avid football player, and reports difficulty in dealing with him due to new onset of anger outbursts. He is noted to have extensive acne and gynecomastia on physical exam. What drugs is he likely abusing?
   a. Marijuana
   b. Methamphetamine
   c. Anabolic steroids
   d. Cocaine

94. Which of the following medications, when given to febrile children, has been linked to the development of Reye's syndrome?
   a. Acetaminophen (Tylenol)
   b. Naprosyn (Aleve)
   c. Aspirin
   d. Ibuprofen (Motrin)

95. On a history form, a nurse practitioner notes that a client has had an enucleation of the eye in the past? What does this consist of?
   a. Removal of the eye
   b. Cataract removal
   c. Retinal repair
   d. Laser vision correction

96. A diabetic client is counseled on the optimum blood pressure for their condition in order to minimize the risk of coronary artery disease. Normal for a diabetic is considered:
   a. 135/85
   b. 140/90
   c. 145/95
   d. 150/95

97. A diabetic client is seen for a clinic visit. What is the urinalysis lab finding that suggests possible kidney damage from the disease process?
    a. Glycosuria
    b. Proteinuria
    c. Hematuria
    d. Low specific gravity

98. As part of standard care for diabetics, which of the following specialists should they see for a yearly consultation?
    a. Psychiatrist
    b. Ophthalmologist
    c. Social Worker
    d. Nephrologist

99. At a yearly health screening exam for a sexually active female, what vaccine should be offered if the client has never received it?
    a. Hepatitis C vaccine
    b. Hepatitis B vaccine
    c. HIV vaccine
    d. MMR booster

100. Which of the followings OTC creams is usually shown to be beneficial in the treatment of adolescent acne?
    a. Aspercreme
    b. Ben-Gay
    c. Bactine
    d. Salicylic acid

101. A 5 year old client has a mild fever and reddened rash on both cheeks, which causes him to have the appearance that he has been slapped. The most likely cause of this is:
    a. Parvovirus B19
    b. Measles
    c. Chicken pox
    d. Mumps

102. A client with recurrent back pain asks a nurse practitioner what exercises would be good for strengthening his lower back and core muscles. All of the following would be good answers *except*:
    a. Tai-chi
    b. Yoga
    c. Pilates
    d. Running

103. Which vaccine that is commonly given in Africa and Asia can lead to false positive reading of Mantoux (PPD) skin tests for TB?
    a. Yellow fever
    b. BCG
    c. MMR
    d. Varicella

104. A client starts a new job using vibratory tools. She reports new onset of tingling on the ventral palms, index finger and middle finger of her dominant hand. This tingling is worse with use and often wakes her at night. What is the most likely cause?
   a. Reynaud's disease
   b. Osteoarthritis
   c. Rheumatoid arthritis
   d. Carpal Tunnel Syndrome

105. A 50 year old female client wishes to prevent osteoporosis. What is the best exercise recommendation in this case?
   a. Water aerobics
   b. Hiking
   c. Biking
   d. Swimming

106. Which of the following GI conditions may also involve the esophagus?
   a. Crohn's disease
   b. Diverticulitis
   c. Diverticulosis
   d. Ulcerative colitis

107. All of the following can cause atrial fibrillation at high doses *except*:
   a. Alcohol
   b. Caffeine
   c. Acetaminophen (Tylenol)
   d. Cocaine

108. Which of the following medications has been shown to be a beneficial treatment for the cessation of smoking?
   a. Methylphenidate (Ritalin)
   b. Naloxone (Narcan)
   c. Butorphanol (Stadol)
   d. Varenicline (Chantix)

109. A pediatric client is noted to have a pruritic scaly rash on the antecubital and popliteal fossas. What is the most likely diagnosis?
   a. Contact dermatitis
   b. Systemic lupus erythematosus (SLE)
   c. Melasma
   d. Eczema

110. A 2 pack per day smoker needs to wear a respirator at his new job as an auto painter. What test is determines his capability for respirator fitness?
   a. Pulmonary function testing (PFT)
   b. ABG
   c. CXR
   d. Treadmill testing

111. A client works as a police officer. His duty station involves the maintenance and upkeep of the shooting range. What blood test should he have done yearly for monitoring occupational exposures?
   a. Arsenic
   b. Lead
   c. Mercury
   d. Thallium

112. A client reports pain anterior to the heel, worse when just arising in the morning and better as the day continues. What is the most likely diagnosis?
   a. Plantar fasciitis
   b. Morton's neuroma
   c. Bunion
   d. Hammertoe

113. A newborn is diagnosed with a heart murmur. This is discovered to be due to a hole between the atria of the heart that did not close. What is this known as?
   a. Patent ductus arteriosus
   b. Patent foramen ovale
   c. Ventricular aneurysm
   d. Mitral valve stenosis

114. An infant has a rash in the groin that is red with numerous "satellite" lesions in the periphery. What is the most likely cause?
   a. Tinea versicolor
   b. Diaper candidiasis
   c. Varicella
   d. Molluscum contagiosum

115. A teenage client with Marfan's syndrome should be screened periodically for what?
   a. Aneurysms
   b. Growth retardation
   c. Hypothyroidism
   d. Colon cancer

116. Which of the following vaccines should not be given to a client with severe egg allergies?
   a. Pneumococcal
   b. Measles
   c. Hepatitis B
   d. Tetanus

117. The Thompson test is used to assess the functionality of what body part?
   a. Quadriceps
   b. Elbow
   c. Shoulder
   d. Achilles tendon

118. Attention deficit disorder is characterized by inattention, distractibility, and impulsivity. Which of the following is NOT one of the criteria used in diagnosing ADD?
    a. Onset of symptoms before age 7
    b. Symptoms must last at least 6 months
    c. Positive family history
    d. Symptoms must be present in at least 2 settings

119. What is the name of the staging system used to measure breast and pubic hair development?
    a. Tanner
    b. Rhomberg
    c. Glasgow
    d. Mallampati

120. A client has been exposed to loud noises due to his occupational and had not worn protective hearing at all times. For what audiological malady is he at risk?
    a. Hearing loss in the low frequency range
    b. Hearing loss in the middle frequency range
    c. Hearing loss in the high frequency range
    d. Loud noise does not cause hearing loss

121. Pediatric clients are routinely monitored for obesity using the Body Mass Index (BMI). This value is found using a chart after first measuring:
    a. Head circumference
    b. Waist circumference
    c. Body fat by calipers
    d. Height and weight

122. An obese pediatric client is suspected of having obstructive sleep apnea syndrome (OSAS). The best diagnostic test for this condition is:
    a. CT of head and neck
    b. Pulse oximetry
    c. Nocturnal polysomnography (sleep study)
    d. Lateral x-ray of neck

123. Arrange the following according to Maslow's hierarchy of human needs from basic to advanced:
    a. Safety
    b. Physiological
    c. Esteem
    d. Self-actualization
    e. 5. Love/Belonging

124. Arrange the following skills for a toddler from the earliest mastered to the latest.
    a. Drink from cup
    b. Wash and dry hands
    c. Smile spontaneously
    d. Prepare cereal

125. Arrange the following gross motor skills for toddlers from the earliest mastered to the latest.
   a. Roll over
   b. Balance on each foot
   c. Sit with no support
   d. Walk up steps

126. A pediatric client is to be given amoxicillin (Amoxil) for an infection. The client weighs 30 Kg and the dosage is 40 mg/kg/day divided tid. What size chewable tablets should they take tid?
   a. 125 mg
   b. 400 mg
   c. 250 mg
   d. 200 mg

127. Which of the following hand lacerations has the highest risk of infection?
   a. Index finger laceration from wooden board contusion
   b. Knee laceration from a hammer
   c. Cheek laceration from fall
   d. Index finger laceration from assaulting another person in the mouth

128. A client comes in to the clinic for an evaluation for a DOT card to be a truck driver. Which of the following medical conditions will preclude the client from passing the test?
   a. Hypothyroidism
   b. Seizure disorder
   c. Hypertension
   d. Finger amputation

129. The follow lab results are received for a patient. Which of the following results are abnormal? Note: More than one answer may be correct.
   a. Hemoglobin 10.4 g/dL.
   b. Total cholesterol 340 mg/dL.
   c. Total serum protein 7.0 g/dL.
   d. Glycosylated hemoglobin A1C 5.4%.

130. The mother of a 14-month-old child reports to the nurse practitioner that her child will not fall asleep at night without a bottle of milk in the crib and often wakes during the night asking for another. Which of the following instructions by the nurse practitioner is correct?
   a. Allow the child to have the bottle at bedtime, but withhold the one later in
   a. the night.
   b. Put juice in the bottle instead of milk.
   c. Give only a bottle of water at bedtime.
   d. Do not allow bottles in the crib.

131. Which of the following actions is NOT appropriate in the care of a 2-month-old infant?
    a. Place the infant on her back for naps and bedtime.
    b. Allow the infant to cry for 5 minutes before responding if she wakes during the night as she may fall back asleep.
    c. Talk to the infant frequently and make eye contact to encourage language development.
    d. Wait until at least 4 months to add infant cereals and strained fruits to the diet.

132. An older patient asks a nurse practitioner to recommend strategies to prevent constipation. Which of the following suggestions would be helpful? Note: More than one answer may be correct.
    a. Get moderate exercise for at least 30 minutes each day.
    b. Drink 6-8 glasses of water each day.
    c. Eat a diet high in fiber.
    d. Take a mild laxative if you don't have a bowel movement every day.

133. Which of the following strategies is NOT effective for prevention of Lyme disease?
    a. Insect repellant on the skin and clothes when in a Lyme endemic area.
    b. Long sleeved shirts and long pants.
    c. Prophylactic antibiotic therapy prior to anticipated exposure to ticks.
    d. Careful examination of skin and hair for ticks following anticipated exposure.

134. A nurse practitioner is counseling patients at a health clinic on the importance of immunizations. Which of the following information is the most accurate regarding immunizations?
    a. All infectious diseases can be prevented with proper immunization.
    b. Immunizations provide natural immunity from disease.
    c. Immunizations are risk-free and should be universally administered.
    d. Immunization provides acquired immunity from some specific diseases.

135. A mother calls the clinic to report that her son has recently started medication to treat attention deficit/hyperactivity disorder (ADHD). The mother fears her son is experiencing side effects of the medicine. Which of the following side effects are typically related to medications used for ADHD? Note: More than one answer may be correct:
    a. Poor appetite.
    b. Insomnia.
    c. Sleepiness.
    d. Agitation.

136. A nurse practitioner is assessing a clinic patient with a diagnosis of hepatitis A. Which of the following is the most likely route of transmission?
    a. Sexual contact with an infected partner.
    b. Contaminated food.
    c. Blood transfusion.
    d. Illegal drug use.

137. A nurse practitioner has diagnosed acute gastritis in a clinic patient. Which of the following medications would be contraindicated for this patient?
   a. Naproxen sodium (Naprosyn).
   b. Calcium carbonate.
   c. Clarithromycin (Biaxin).
   d. Furosemide (Lasix).

138. A nonimmunized child appears at the clinic with a visible rash. Which of the following observations indicates the child may have rubeola (measles)?
   a. Small blue-white spots are visible on the oral mucosa.
   b. The rash begins on the trunk and spreads outward.
   c. There is low-grade fever.
   d. The lesions have a "tear drop on a rose petal" appearance.

139. A child weighing 30 kg arrives at the clinic with diffuse itching as the result of an allergic reaction to an insect bite. Diphenhydramine (Benadryl) 25 mg 3 times a day is prescribed. The correct pediatric dose is 5 mg/kg/day. Which of the following best describes the prescribed drug dose?
   a. It is the correct dose.
   b. The dose is too low.
   c. The dose is too high.
   d. The dose should be increased or decreased, depending on the symptoms.

140. The mother of a 2-month-old infant brings the child to the clinic for a well baby check. She is concerned because she feels only one testis in the scrotal sac. Which of the following statements about the undescended testis is the most accurate?
   a. Normally, the testes are descended by birth.
   b. The infant will likely require surgical intervention.
   c. The infant probably has with only one testis.
   d. Normally, the testes descend by one year of age.

141. An adolescent brings a physician's note to school stating that he is not to participate in sports due to a diagnosis of Osgood-Schlatter disease. Which of the following statements about the disease is correct?
   a. The condition was caused by the student's competitive swimming schedule.
   b. The student will most likely require surgical intervention.
   c. The student experiences pain in the inferior aspect of the knee.
   d. The student is trying to avoid participation in physical education.

142. The nurse practitioner asks a 13-year-old female to bend forward at the waist with arms hanging freely. Which of the following assessments is the nurse most likely conducting?
   a. Spinal flexibility.
   b. Leg length disparity.
   c. Hypostatic blood pressure.
   d. Scoliosis.

143. A child with chronic bronchial asthma tells the nurse practitioner she is asking for a puppy for Christmas. The child's mother asks if pets are advisable for a child with this condition. Which of the following responses is the most appropriate?
    a. Pets with hair or feathers are likely to trigger asthma attacks.
    b. It's all right to get the child a dog, as long as it's a short -haired breed.
    c. A cat would be a better pet for this child.
    d. It's all right to get the child a dog, as long as it doesn't sleep in the child's bed.

144. Non-steroidal anti-inflammatory drugs (NSAIDs) are used to relieve pain and treat musculoskeletal inflammation. Which of the following information about NSAIDs is important for patients to understand?
    a. NSAIDs can cause irreversible liver damage if taken in excessive doses.
    b. Serum levels of NSAID medications need not remain therapeutic to have an anti-inflammatory effect.
    c. NSAIDs can irritate the stomach lining and should be taken with food.
    d. NSAIDs should be taken every 4 hours for pain relief.

145. An infant is born with flat facies, a single palmar crease, low-set ears, and hypotonia. Which of the following conditions is most likely the cause of these abnormalities?
    a. Trisomy 21.
    b. Trisomy 13.
    c. Fetal alcohol syndrome.
    d. In utero rubella infection.

146. A patient is trying to lower her blood pressure by modifying her lifestyle. Which of the following is an appropriate lifestyle change to help lower her blood pressure?
    a. Starting atenolol (Tenormin), a beta-blocker.
    b. Losing weight.
    c. Increasing leisure activities.
    d. Beginning a vegetarian diet.

147. A 15-month-old has severe diaper dermatitis. Which of the following approaches is the most beneficial?
    a. Minimize diaper changes to avoid irritating the area.
    b. Clean the area frequently with baby wipes.
    c. Begin toilet training as soon as possible.
    d. Clean the area with water and mild soap and dry thoroughly.

148. A morbidly obese patient wants to lose weight and asks a nurse practitioner about surgical weight loss options. Which of the following information is the most accurate?
    a. Weight loss surgery is recommended for patients who are 50 lbs. or more overweight.
    b. Gastric banding has a higher risk profile than gastric bypass.
    c. Weight loss surgery is recommended for patients with a body mass index (BMI) of 40 or greater.
    d. Weight loss surgery is more effective than other weight loss programs.

149. A nurse practitioner is evaluating an overweight patient for type 2 diabetes. Which of the following symptoms is NOT a sign of type 2 diabetes?
   a. Increased thirst.
   b. Increased urination.
   c. Blurred vision.
   d. Loss of appetite.

150. A 2-month-old infant is scheduled to receive immunizations at his well baby visit. Which of the following vaccines should the nurse practitioner prepare for administration?
   a. Diphtheria, tetanus, and acellular pertussis (DTaP) #1, hepatitis B (HepB) #1, and inactivated poliovirus (IPV) #1.
   b. DTaP #1, HepB #2, and oral polio vaccine (OPV) #1
   c. DTaP #1, HepB #1, OPV #1, and Haemophilus b #1.
   d. HepB #1, IPV #1, and measles, mumps, rubella (MMR).

Answer Key and Explanations

1. C: Albuterol is a bronchodilator, which is given first, to open the airway. Flovent is a corticosteroid, which decreases the inflammation, followed by Tobramycin, which is an antibiotic. Giving the antibiotic last ensures that the maximum amount of medication can be absorbed.

2. A: Specific, open-ended questions about what is going on currently with the patient, as well as questions about past medical history, help to prioritize immediate needs and concerns and to make the appropriate interventions and referrals. The other information listed in b, c, and d can be answered at a later time.

3. B: A patient with flank pain, even though it has been two days, may have a blockage from a kidney stone, which requires immediate pain relief and workup. The three-year-old with vomiting should be next due to the concern for dehydration and to rule out causes for the vomiting. The infant with a fever, even though smiling, should be seen next for possible medications to control the fever, followed by the man with the nail.

4. D: is the most appropriate subtle symptom, which should alert the nurse practitioner that this is a change in condition and a signal that the child has been compensating due to some illness and now is worse. This child should be seen to rule out head injury, meningitis, and a variety of other possible illnesses.

5. C: is the most appropriate when discussing this over the phone. You are not able to visualize and assess the patient, so an immediate evaluation is warranted to rule out an impending stroke or brain bleed. The 24- to 48-hour suggestion negates the seriousness of what may be happening; you can't assume it is alcohol or lack of sleep from the information given, and answer d may take too long or may be forgotten.

6. D: is the most appropriate. The nurse practitioner should recognize that women do not always have classic chest pain symptoms or break out in a sweat when having a myocardial infarction. Bilateral elbow pain, low blood pressure, and low heart rate may indicate a heart attack, which should be ruled out quickly to get the patient to the appropriate facility.

7. A: is the most appropriate nonverbal indication for any age patient who is experiencing difficulty breathing. Sweating is not the first sign of respiratory distress in a healthy patient, and slight wheezing may be normal for some patients when lifting.

8. B: is most appropriate. In the clinic, it is most important to get to the current complaint and what led up to the problem to best quickly assess what interventions may be needed. Past medical and surgical history are important but not before finding out what the current complaint is. Current medications and allergies are the next important thing to know during an assessment in order to make an accurate assessment and an appropriate plan or intervention.

9. C: is most appropriate. You can never assume a patient has a low pain tolerance, and it is not wise to give oral fluids or food to a patient until after evaluating him or her. A patient with clammy, pale skin and an irregular heart rate should never be placed in the waiting room.

10. C: is the most appropriate way to ask a patient if they feel safe or if they are ever afraid. Asking in front of the possible abuser will never result in an honest answer due to the patient's fear. It is mandatory in most states that the nurse practitioner must ask about abuse, so it should never be ignored. Describing your own experience is not appropriate or professional.

11. B: would be the most appropriate for a teenager with fruity breath and sleepiness. The urine dipstick may show whether ketones are being spilled into the urine, and the glucometer will give an immediate blood glucose level. The clinician can then use this information to determine if diabetes is suspected or if another avenue of diagnosis should be pursued. Positive ketones and high blood glucose levels would indicate that the teen should be further evaluated for diabetes. Rapid strep tests are appropriate for the ambulatory care setting but would not be the first, quick, on-site laboratory test ordered for this teen.

12. C: is most appropriate. Rapid streptococcal throat cultures are available in the office setting and provide the clinician a quick diagnostic tool to help get patients started on antibiotics sooner. The test is to provide the best care possible for the patient and not to protect the liability of the facility or to protect the staff from the patient. Providing another reason to bill would not be a valid reason to do these tests in the outpatient setting.

13. D: is the most appropriate. A respiratory nebulizer treatment would be the invasive treatment of choice to assist this patient with wheezing and shortness of breath. Blood pressure monitoring is noninvasive and would be part of the assessment, but a urine dipstick and blood glucose monitoring are not immediately needed with a complaint of wheezing.

14. A: is the most appropriate. Vision exams are part of most kindergarten exams and can be done in the office setting. Immunizations are invasive, strep tests are not routine for a kindergarten physical, and occult blood tests are not routine, either. Occult blood tests are most often done for adults.

15. D: is the most appropriate. It is not appropriate to turn a patient away without a full assessment exam and history. Most states allow an 18-year-old to be treated without parental permission, but, regardless, a patient is not turned away. Minor children may require the nurse practitioner to call for parental permission, depending on the policy at your facility. The nurse practitioner will always treat the patient with dignity and protect his or her privacy while preparing the patient for the examinations necessary to properly diagnose the symptoms.

16. A: is most appropriate. On-site testing is convenient for the patient, offers early diagnosis and prevention, and is cost-effective, especially when it prevents hospitalization. It does bring in revenue for the facility but does not give the facility the ability to test all patients just for the sake of bringing in cash. There is a financial advantage when tests are

ordered for appropriate patients. Answer d is incorrect; there is no data that support lab results being inaccurate in an office etting.

17. B: is the most likely result of improper disinfection. Patient safety is always one of the prime purposes of cleanliness and disinfection. Room air does not destroy all bacteria, so sterilization and disinfection are mandatory in any health-care facility. No other data are needed to make an appropriate choice here.

18. B: is the most appropriate answer. A peak flow meter can help to determine how much respiratory distress a teen is in and gives the nurse an idea about how the child is compensating. A chest X-ray may be ordered after the physician has examined the patient or after a low reading on the peak flow meter to determine if there is an underlying infection. Blood glucose levels and drug screens are not routine exams when evaluating for wheezing.

19. A: is the statement that demonstrates the nurse practitioner practicing primary prevention by discussing seat belt safety and safety with car seat restraints. These are preventative measures that parents can be taught to reduce injuries in young children. Answer b shows hospitality but does not demonstrate prevention. Performing an assessment is an appropriate skill but is not considered prevention. Documentation is a responsibility of the nurse practitioner, but the statement does not include education, which may be considered prevention.

20. B: is the statement that clearly shows that secondary prevention involves education regarding early diagnosis and prompt treatment for any condition. The other choices do not demonstrate the definition of secondary prevention.

21. C: is the client who would respond best to consistent follow up with the same staff in an office care setting, which could provide continuity of care and support for a teen whose mother works. The continuity would help with the consistent assessment, education, and implementation of the treatment plan. A new mom with a healthy newborn may not have any bad effects from seeing a different physician or provider or not following up as suggested. An elderly diabetic who lives with her daughter is getting consistent care from a family member and may not be seen on a consistent basis in the office setting. A toddler with chicken pox may or may not be followed up in an office setting.

22. B: Chronically ill clients still need wellness education to prevent further complications and to prevent acute illness. Answer a is incorrect, answer c is inappropriate, and the cost of a chronic illness is increased, so education and prevention will help to decrease further costs in acute illness.

23. C: Statements a and b show the nurse practitioner offering outside resources for a client. Answer d is incorrect and limiting.

24. C: The nurse practitioner knows that different illnesses are reimbursed differently and that wellness care is reimbursed at a different rate then acute illness. Wellness care may be very cost-effective, so prevention and education are part of the nurse practitioner's responsibility when planning client care. The nurse practitioner doesn't need an accounting degree to understand the cost of care and to implement cost-effective ways to give care. Case management is very cost-effective in most cases and is implemented in office setting.

25. D: is the correct category of care management when the nurse practitioner is referring a patient for further education outside of the office care setting.

26. B: Critical pathways give specific interventions and measurable outcomes for the health-care team, allowing them to evaluate each patient with a certain list of symptoms and expected results against unexpected or bad results. Payroll doesn't directly relate to performance improvement, but the payroll department would have their own set of performance criteria. Marketing brochures and staff schedules also do not directly relate to patient interventions and outcomes.

27. C: In the office care setting where a patient may only be seen occasionally, it is important for the health-care team to relate important information to the client's other physicians, especially relating to an ongoing health issue and acute symptoms. Answer a is incorrect, and b is partially correct because the nurse practitioner would make sure that the physician understood the client's medical history. Answer d is also incorrect.

28. A: The Internet allows the nurse practitioner to look up diseases, medications, and addresses and get locations or phone information to meet the needs of the client. The Internet should not be used as a distraction for when the patient load is light. Ordering meals for personal consumption is not a reason to access the Internet while working in the office care setting.

29. B: is most appropriate for part of the treatment plan. A return appointment may be needed but doesn't help solve the domestic abuse problem. Community resources offer places to find solutions and alternatives for the client. A job or work program may be part of the answer, but the question doesn't give enough information for this to be a resource that can be part of the treatment. The police department would be a community resource to report the abuse to but not a place that would offer alternatives and treatments. Answer b is more related to the types of resources that would help in the long term in solving the issue of domestic violence.

30. C: The nurse practitioner must be prepared for the client who takes a turn or who may be more ill than first thought. The facility should have protocols in place for the transfer and referral to an acute care facility or specialty hospital in the case of an emergency. Any client who appears to be getting worse should be reassessed and treated before taking care of the other clients in the clinic. Reassessment should occur, but that does not take the intervention far enough in the case of a critical child. Children compensate for a time, but when a child shows critical changes, they must be acted upon. A child appearing to get worse during the clinic visit may not be sent home, depending on the symptoms.

31. B: Occasional blood may not need treatment but should never be overlooked without an evaluation. Blood does not always indicate infection. It could indicate a kidney or bladder stone, trauma, or inflammation. Male clients do present with blood in their urine.

32. A: Although the nurse practitioner may provide mechanisms to measure patient satisfaction and access to care as well as continuity of care, with the information given, patient education would be the most appropriate answer. Education regarding the cessation of smoking should be given regardless of the treatment or outcome for the shortness of breath.

33. B: As a patient advocate in the office care setting, it is part of the nurse practitioner's role to make certain the proper referral is made and the right provider and level of care are given.

34. A: The facility should have policies on how to deal with complaints, how to resolve them, and to improve things in the future. This data will help determine client satisfaction and what kind of job the facility is doing. Answer b is incorrect. Answer c is not correct because the end result of a client diagnosis and treatment may be great, and the client satisfaction may still be low, making the end result unrelated. Answer d is also not correct either and is not a reliable source of evaluation.

35. D: is the most appropriate for advocating for the client. The other skills are an asset to being an nurse practitioner, but answer d is most related to being a patient advocate. The other skills do make the facility run more smoothly and efficiently.

36. A: As an advocate for the client, it is important that the nurse practitioner provides options for care and gives enough information so the client can make informed decisions regarding their health care. Answers b and c are not correct. Answer d does not demonstrate how the nurse advocates for the client.

37. B: would be the most appropriate concern for the nurse practitioner.

38. C: The nurse practitioner is more likely to get the true answers if the client is questioned in private and away from the possible assailant. Continuing to question in front of the companion may not result in honest answers, and accusing the client will add to her fear. The nurse practitioner must report child abuse, but it is not always advisable to report suspected domestic violence without further probing.

39. D: All of the answer choices will assist the nurse practitioner in keeping open communication between team members and reducing conflict in the workplace.

40. B: Identifying, and then avoiding, gestures that may be offensive shows respect for other cultures. A nurse practitioner should never disregard a client's desire for modesty. Failing to modify communication patterns may fail to properly inform or educate a client, and failing to use clarifying techniques forces the nurse practitioner to assume the client understands when maybe the client is misinterpreting the information.

41. C: "Space" refers to the physical distance occurring in personal interactions including personal, intimate, and public contacts. Different cultures react differently to this type of distance. Knowing how people of a certain culture feel about space during a personal interaction will guide the nurse practitioner in meeting the needs of the client in a comfortable way. Answers a, b, and d are not correct.

42. A: Although the other answers may have a minimal impact on the way a client reacts to what is being said, the socioeconomic and educational levels of a client have the most influence on how the client perceives what is being said.

43. B: Avoidance and ignorance do nothing for enhancing the care of a client. A translator may not be necessary for many cultures, but respect is universal in enhancing relationships and the care of the client.

44. C: A translator would ensure that the client and the family understood the instructions. Hand gestures and return demonstration would not ensure that the client understood the medication and side effects.

45. B: Often there are local or community resources or support groups that will assist a client with financial needs. The other answers are not appropriate.

46. A: Reporting from one facility to the other is one responsibility the nurse practitioner must assume. The other statements are not correct. Other team members may be involved, but communication between the sending facility and the accepting facility should rest with the nurse practitioner caring for the client.

47. B: In most facilities, it is necessary to have a fax cover sheet, along with a release of information signed by the client. This protects the privacy of the client and will specifically list the items being requested. A cover sheet alone will not be enough. A signed release should always be accompanied by a cover sheet or letterhead from the facility making the request. A phone call may speed up the process, but the facility releasing the information should never release anything without a signed release first, proving the information is being requested by an appropriate facility.

48. C: A telephone log can be as simple as a spiral notebook indicating the date, time, and information offered to the caller. A note can be made in the patient chart on paper or in the computer. Some simple telephone encounters may not require written documentation, depending on the policies of the facility, especially calls that give out standard information such as business hours or a simple inquiry about services offered. Telephone encounters that must be documented are related to patient complaints, the plan of care offered, and the patient's agreement or disagreement with what action should be taken next. It is important to document what the patient verbalizes as a way to make clear what it is they understood about the plan.

49. B: Documentation should be concise but must always include all aspects of what has happened with the care of the client for legal reasons.

50. B: It is never professional to discuss another client's diagnosis, regardless of whether the clients are friends or not. Ignoring the question does not establish the professional boundary that should be set by the nurse practitioner . It is never professional to discuss the information in generic terms, either, because this still crosses the professional boundaries established to protect the privacy of clients treated at the clinic.

51. C: Hospice will have a social services team member who will work with the family to find the appropriate end-of-life care for this client as well as nurses, physicians, and spiritual support. Social services alone may also be helpful but may be more time consuming than going directly to hospice. The oncologist referral would most likely already be in place because of the diagnosis, and speech therapy would not be a top priority at this point in time.

52. A: There should be a policy in place when assessing a client with suicidal thoughts or feelings long before such a patient would appear at the clinic. An appropriate way to assess, report, and protect the patient should be determined for consistent and professional treatment of any suicidal client. Notifying the police would not be appropriate initially.

Documentation is important, but it would be a team effort in deciding treatment. The nurse practitioner would discuss the client's complaints but should be mentally forming a plan of action, depending on the policy of the facility.

53. D: Education may include dietary suggestions, how to monitor a fluid intake diary, and Kegel exercises to strengthen pelvic muscles in an effort to decrease urinary incontinence. Medications, referrals to surgeons, and diagnostic testing may fall within the scope of practice for nurse practitioners, depending on the state and on their education. However, under most circumstances, answer d is most correct and within the scope of practice and professional boundaries of the basic nurse practitioner.

54. D: This would not be an example of good leadership. It is important to promote standards of care, to be an example for new nurse practitioners, and to encourage shared governance. Encouraging the importance of certification and validating the team members who become certified are an important part of leadership.

55. C: The U.S. Department of Labor and the Occupational Safety and Health Administration regulate the standards and rules for safety in the workplace.

56. C: The Centers for Disease Control and Prevention (CDC) offers regulations and standards of care for contagious diseases, especially those that can cause a pandemic. The ADA offers standards for diabetes, the AHA offers standards for heart disease and prevention, and OSHA regulates workplace safety.

57. B: Confidentiality is part of patient safety. Falls are part of patient safety goals in every setting. Side effects of medications are part of patient safety in every setting and include side effects, right dose, right time, right patient, right route, and right medication. There are national patient safety goals mandating the standard of safe patient care.

58. C: The common procedure codes allow providers to use the same code for the most common procedures, making it easier for reimbursement for those services. While jobs are created, that is not the purpose for the system. It does allow for consistency in classifications, but errors in coding will still occur due to human error.

59. D: The other choices are not real.

60. B: Those are all examples of health-care delivery systems with different plans for reimbursement.

61. C: The endpoint is always that the care delivered made a difference and when it doesn't, the delivery of care must be reevaluated and changed so it will make a difference. The other three choices are not true.

62. D: All of the statements improve performance and outcomes in the short term and long term for patient outcomes.

63. C: It would be most appropriate to offer diet and nutrition, exercise, and weight management education in the course of assessing and treating the child. Developing a rapport with a teen by asking appropriate questions regarding favorite foods, favorite activities, and the health hazards of obesity can all be discussed in a nonthreatening way

and can help to educate the child and parent on weight management. Opening the discussion can give the nurse the opportunity to make a referral to a dietitian or exercise program as well.

64. A: Material must be age appropriate and applicable to the patient. The other choices are not correct; graphic education may be offensive and so may be material that is not sensitive to culture. Reading material is not always appropriate, depending on the reading level of the patient.

65. D: All those factors will determine how to present the information on smoking and its hazards and the process of cessation. Community programs can be modified to better meet the needs of those in attendance.

66. D: When educating a group in the community, the grade level and mental development level of the group will indicate the level of difficulty the material can be presented at. In the case of teens, parental consent or teacher input should also be considered when giving educational information of a sexual nature, such as pregnancy prevention.

67. A: It is never too late to modify diet and exercise habits to prevent or halt heart disease. The other three choices are incorrect information and should not be shared.

68. B: Asthma can be managed, and compliance is essential. It is a serious illness if not managed and can be fatal. Inhalers must be taken in the right order to be effective. The bronchodilator is first to open the airway, followed by the steroids. Rinsing the mouth after inhaling steroids will help to prevent thrush.

69. B: The classic presentation for pyloric stenosis is refractory projectile emesis in a first born male infant at around 6 weeks of age. Confirmation of diagnosis is performed with ultrasound of the abdomen which finds an enlargement of the pylorus. This is treated with operative intervention.

70. D: The use of antibiotics in the past six weeks is a risk factor for *Clostridium difficile*. Antibiotic use disrupts the normal flora of the bowel leading to overgrowth by *C. difficile* with the release of toxins and resulting in inflammation.

71. A: Answers 2, 3, and 4 are all first line treatments for constipation in the elderly. Stimulant laxatives should be avoided as they can lead to dependence and irregularity in the gastrointestinal tract.

72. B: If given in the third trimester, NSAID medication can cause premature closure of the ductus arteriosus of the fetus and should be avoided. The other treatments are all acceptable.

73. C: Although use of the varicella vaccine is now widespread, it is still common. An annoyance in most patients, it can be life-threatening in immunocompromised patients such as those on chemotherapy, radiation, or with HIV/AIDS.

74. A: LDL is the prominent "bad" cholesterol and is the strongest predictor for future coronary artery disease. It needs to be as low as possible and the acceptable level for LDL depends on the number of risk factors the client has.

75. D: Prolonged sitting during long trips is thought to be a risk factor for DVT. The other activities may help prevent this.

76. C: Any kind of liquid that contains sugars can cause dental caries if given in a bottle at nighttime.

77. B: In bilingual households, children usually develop speech slightly later due to the assimilation of two languages, but by school age there is no difference.

78. C: Carbonated sodas alkalinize the urine and may impair the clearance of bacteria. Cranberry juice and extract acidify the urine and prevent adhesion of bacteria to the bladder wall. Pyridium acts as an analgesic.

79. C: A decreased peak flow is the most reliable indicator that asthma may be worsening. It is therefore vital that the client's family know what the baseline is so that any deviation can be quickly addressed.

80. C: Accutane is a vitamin A derivative that is very beneficial in treatingcystic type acne. It can cause severe birth defects if given during pregnancy so two forms of birth control are needed during treatment.

81. A: Keeping eyelids open can help prevent gagging with any swabbing of the throat.

82. A: In order to minimize contaminants, blood cultures are taken from the antecubital fossa after sterilizing with iodine and using sterile gloves.

83. C: For a PPD (Mantoux) skin test, the clients arm must be examined between 48 to 72 hours later.

84. C: Tegaderm bandages are used for skin tears and should be left on for 2 to 3 days until seen again by the practitioner.

85. B: Carbonated beverages can exacerbate GERD and should beminimized as much as possible. Decreasing caffeine, alcohol, and weight are all appropriate.

86. A: Lasix is a diuretic that does not require any monitoring of blood levels. Digoxin and lithium both require monitoring for their blood levels and warfarin requires monitoring of the bleeding time.

87. C: Rice is a carbohydrate and is not high in iron. Spinach and meats are high in this element.

88. A: Intrauterine devices (IUDs) are effective in preventing pregnancy but have no action against the spread of HPV or other STDs.

89. A: Smoking increases the risk of DVT and heart disease in women taking oral contraceptive pills. Smokers should be offered other choices first.

90. A: The use of laxatives for weight control is a sign of possible bulimia and this usage should prompt further investigation. The other responses are common to most clients in the teenage years.

91. C: The act of returning to behaviors of a prior age is regression. Repression involves sublimating anxieties, rationalization involves explaining objectionable behaviors, and transference involves projection of feelings onto others.

92. D: If uncorrected, undescended testes have an increased risk of cancer in later life. If not descended by early childhood it is recommended that they have surgical correction.

93. C: Emotional outbursts, rapid muscular weight gain, acne, and gynecomastia are common manifestations of anabolic steroid abuse. Abuse by high school athletes is unfortunately very common and can lead to long term side effects.

94. C: Aspirin has been linked as the causative agent of Reye's syndrome. It should not be used as an anti-pyretic in febrile children under the age of 18.

95. A: Enucleation involves the complete removal of the eye. It is usually performed after severe trauma or cancer.

96. A: Although 140/90 may be considered normal for most in the population, 135/85 is considered the upper limit of normal for diabetics.

97. B: The initial finding on urinalysis, which is indicative of damage to the kidneys from diabetes, is proteinuria. Glycosuria and hematuria are worrisome findings but not direct findings of kidney damage from diabetes.

98. B: As part of standard diabetic care, diabetics should have a yearly dilated eye exam by an ophthalmologist to ensure no retinopathy is developing. Those diabetics with kidney involvement may need referrals to the nephrologist but not all diabetics will.

99. B: If not already done, the client should be offered the Hepatitis B vaccine series to prevent the disease. A vaccine for Hepatitis C and HIV does not exist and the MMR series should have been done in childhood.

100. D: Creams with salicylic acid can be beneficial in the treatment of acne. The creams decrease the bacteria the exacerbate acne and reduce inflammation. The other answers are used for musculoskeletal issues.

101. A: Parvovirus B19 causes "fifth's disease", a viral illness characterized by a fever and a "slapped cheek" rash. It is self-limiting but it is important to note that transmission to a fetus is detrimental and those infected should be sheltered from anyone pregnant.

102. D: Although a good aerobic exercise, running is not an exercise that will greatly increase lower back and core strength like the other answers will.

103. B: The BCG (Bacillus Calmette-Guerin) vaccine is given in many developing countries, and this can lead to false positive reading with PPD skin tests.

104. D: The symptoms listed and the new onset of work with a vibratory tool are all classic for carpal tunnel syndrome. After conservative treatment if the symptoms persist, testing with an electromyelogram (EMG) may be needed.

105. B: The most important exercises used for osteoporosis prevention are weight bearing exercises. Hiking is the only weight bearing exercise listed.

106. A: Crohn's disease can involve any part of the digestive system from mouth to anus. The other answers are all limited to the colon.

107. C: In high doses, Tylenol does not greatly increase the risk of atrial fibrillation. The other answers all are known to increase the risk of arrhythmias at high doses.

108. D: Chantix is a non-nicotine prescription medication that has been shown to be beneficial in helping clients with tobacco abuse.

109. D: The antecubital and popliteal fossa are the classic sites for eczema. The rashes of SLE and melasma are usually seen on the face.

110. A: The ability to use a respirator safely, is determined by examination of PFT results. Very low levels of lung function may preclude safe use of a respirator.

111. B: Any client with long term exposure in places that lead may be aerosolized should be monitored for lead poisoning. This would include foundries, shooting ranges, and some factories.

112. A: Pain just anterior to the heel that improves as the day progresses is consistent with plantar fasciitis, an inflammation in the connective tissue on the bottom of the foot. NSAIDs, ice, and stretching may be beneficial.

113. B: A patent foramen ovale is the non-closure of an embryonic component of the heart. Depending on size, surgical correction may be necessary.

114. B: Candidiasis or yeast infection is characterized in children by these "satellite" red lesions in the periphery.

115. A: Tall stature, ophthalmic issues, and the possible development of aortic aneurysms characterize Marfan's syndrome. Clients should have regular screenings.

116. B: Clients with severe egg allergy should avoid measles vaccine, since it is grown on chick fibroblast cells.

117. D: The Thompson test consists of squeezing a client's calf while they are in the prone position to assess for Achilles tendon rupture. An intact tendon will result in extension of the foot.

118. C: Although a positive family history often occurs, it is not a requisite part of the diagnosis. The other answers all must be met to make criteria for the disorder.

119. A: The Tanner staging system is used to classify breast and pubic hair development.

120. C: Long term exposure to loud noises causes hearing loss in the high frequency hearing range. Any exposure over 85 decibels should necessitate hearing protection.

121. D: The BMI is a useful number for analysis of obesity. It is based on a table of height and weight measurements. Although not always accurate in very muscular men due to muscle mass, it is a very quick and easy way to gauge weight loss and gain.

122. C: A sleep study is the gold standard for evaluation of OSAS. The clientis monitored for abnormalities in ventilation and sleep. This condition may benefit from weight loss and CPAP.

123. Answer: 2, 1, 5, 3, 4 is the correct listing of human needs according to Maslow. These start from the most basic animalistic needs up to the most psychological.

124. Answer: 3, 1, 2, 4, is the proper order of social milestone development.

125. Answer: 1, 3, 4, 2 is the proper order of development of gross motor skills.

126. B: If the client weighs 30 Kg and the dose is 40 mg/kg /day, they should take 30 x 40 = 1200 mg/day. If the dose is divided tid it is 1200 mg/ 3 = 400 mg tid.

127. D: Lacerations to the hands occurring from assaults are known as "fight bites" and due to exposure to bacteria from the mouth, have a very high incidence of infection. They all need to be treated with antibiotics and may need inpatient IV therapy.

128. B: Seizure disorder is a limiting condition and clients must be free of seizures for 10 years without the use of medications before they can pass the test.

129. A and B: Normal hemoglobin in adults is 12 – 16 g/dL. Total cholesterol levels of 200 mg/dL or below are considered normal. Total serum protein of 7.0-g/dL and glycosylated hemoglobin A1c of 5.4% are both normal levels.

130. C: Babies and toddlers should not fall asleep with bottles containing liquid other than plain water due to the risk of dental decay. Sugars in milk or juice remain in the mouth during sleep and cause caries, even in teeth that have not yet erupted. When water is substituted for milk or juice, babies will often lose interest in the bottle at night.

131. B: Infants under 6 months may not be able to sleep for long periods because their stomachs are too small to hold adequate nourishment to take them through the night. After 6 months, it may be helpful to let babies put themselves back to sleep after waking during the night, but not prior to 6 months. Infants should always be placed on their backs to sleep. Research has shown a dramatic decrease in sudden infant death syndrome (SIDS) with back sleeping. Eye contact and verbal engagement with infants are important to language development. The best diet for infants under 4 months of age is breast milk or infant formula.

132. A, B, and C: A daily bowel movement is not necessary if the patient is comfortable and the bowels move regularly. Moderate exercise, such as walking, encourages bowel health, as does generous water intake. A diet high in fiber is also helpful.). Laxatives should be used as

a last resort and should not be taken regularly. Over time, laxatives can desensitize the bowel and worsen constipation.

133. C: Prophylactic use of antibiotics is not indicated to prevent Lyme disease. Antibiotics are used only when symptoms develop following a tick bite. Insect repellant should be used on skin and clothing when exposure is anticipated. Clothing should be designed to cover as much exposed area as possible to provide an effective barrier. Close examination of skin and hair can reveal the presence of a tick before a bite occurs.

134. D: Immunization is available for the prevention of some, but not all, specific diseases. This type of immunity is "acquired" by causing antibodies to form in response to a specific pathogen. Natural immunity is present at birth because the infant acquires maternal antibodies Immunization, like all medication, cannot be risk-free and should be considered based on the risk of the disease in question.

135. A, B, and C: ADHD in children is frequently treated with CNS stimulant medications, which increase focus and improve concentration. Children often experience insomnia, agitation, and decreased appetite. Sleepiness is not a side effect of stimulants.

136. B: Hepatitis A is the only type that is transmitted by the fecal-oral route through contaminated food. Hepatitis B, C, and D are transmitted through infected bodily fluids.

137. A: Naproxen sodium is a nonsteroidal anti-inflammatory drug that can cause inflammation of the upper GI tract. For this reason, it is contraindicated in a patient with gastritis. Calcium carbonate is used as an antacid for the relief of indigestion and is not contraindicated. Clarithromycin is an antibacterial often used for the treatment of *Helicobacter pylori* in gastritis. Furosemide is a loop diuretic and is contraindicated in a patient with gastritis.

138. A: Koplik's spots are small blue-white spots visible on the oral mucosa and are characteristic of measles infection. The body rash typically begins on the face and travels downward. High fever is often present. "Tear drop on a rose petal" refers to the lesions found in varicella (chicken pox).

139. B: This child weighs 30 kg, and the pediatric dose of diphenhydramine is 5 mg/kg/day (5 X 30 = 150/day). Therefore, the correct dose is 150 mg/day. Divided into 3 doses per day, the child should receive 50 mg 3 times a day rather than 25 mg 3 times a day.

140. D: Normally, the testes descend by one year of age. In young infants, it is common for the testes to retract into the inguinal canal when the environment is cold or the cremasteric reflex is stimulated. Exam should be done in a warm room with warm hands. It is most likely that both testes are present and will descend by a year. If not, a full assessment will determine the appropriate treatment.

141. C: Osgood-Schlatter disease occurs in adolescents in rapid growth phase when the infrapatellar ligament of the quadriceps muscle pulls on the tibial tubercle, causing pain and swelling in the inferior aspect of the knee. Osgood- Schlatter disease is commonly caused by activities that require repeated use of the quadriceps, including track and soccer. Swimming is not a likely cause. The condition is usually self-limited, responding to ice, rest, and analgesics. Continued participation will worsen the condition and the symptoms.

142. D: A check for scoliosis, a lateral deviation of the spine, is an important part of the routine adolescent exam. It is assessed by having the teen bend at the waist with arms dangling, while observing for lateral curvature and uneven rib level. Scoliosis is more common in female adolescents. Choices A, B, and C are not part of the routine adolescent exam.

143. A: It is important to try to allergy-proof the home of a child with bronchial asthma. Pets with long or short hair or feathers are especially likely to trigger attacks. Cats may be the most frequent cause of pet-induced allergy response.

144. C: NSAIDs can irritate the gastric mucosa and should be taken with food. Acetaminophen (Tylenol) can cause irreversible liver damage in excessive doses, but this is not a characteristic of NSAIDs. NSAIDs should be taken at approximately 6-8 hour intervals to maintain a therapeutic serum level and have the maximum anti-inflammatory effect. A dosing interval of 4 hours is too frequent.

145. A: Trisomy 21, or Down syndrome, causes characteristic anomalies, including up-slanted eyes with an epicanthal fold, flat facies, a palmar crease, abnormally low-set ears, and hypotonia. Trisomy 13 can cause more severe anomalies, such as cleft palate, microcephaly, skeletal abnormalities, and often results in fetal death. Fetal alcohol syndrome is characterized by facial abnormalities, mental retardation, and growth retardation. Congenital rubella typically causes cataracts, deafness, and mental retardation.

146. B: Losing weight is likely to be the most effective lifestyle change for lowering blood pressure. Starting antihypertensive medication such as atenolol is not considered lifestyle change. Increasing leisure activities may improve quality of life, but won't necessarily reduce blood pressure. A vegetarian diet by itself has not been shown to lower blood pressure.

147. D: Severe diaper rash may be difficult to treat in toddlers. It is best to clean the area with water and mild soap, and rinse and dry thoroughly. If the area can be left open to air it may be helpful. The child should not sit in a wet or soiled diaper, as this is very irritating to tender skin. Baby wipes can be irritating due to perfumes and additives. Toddlers should not begin toilet training until they're able to control bowel movements, usually starting around 24 months.

148. C: Weight loss (bariatric) surgery is recommended for very obese patients who are 90 lbs. or more overweight with a body mass index of 40 or greater. It should be considered only after other weight loss programs have failed. Gastric banding procedures generally have a lower risk profile than gastric bypass procedures and are performed laparoscopically. Surgical weight loss is initially very effective but has a significant rate of long-term weight re-gain and associated complications.

149. D: Increased thirst and increased urination are classic signs of the onset of type 2 diabetes. Loss of fluid is the result of osmotic diuresis due to glycosuria. Blurred vision can also occur due to osmotic changes. Increased appetite rather than loss of appetite is also a symptom. Because type 2 diabetes develops slowly, it is common for patients to notice no symptoms initially.

150. A: Infants typically receive their first set of immunizations at the 2-month well baby visit. These include diphtheria, tetanus, and acellular pertussis, hepatitis B, and inactivated poliovirus. Oral polio vaccine is no longer used routinely. Haemophilus B and measles, mumps, rubella vaccines are not given at the 2-month visit.

Practice Test #3

Practice Questions

1. An adult patient needs treatment for *Chlamydia trachomatis* urethritis. Which one of the following drugs is useful as a single-dose regimen?
   a. Ceftriaxone intramuscularly
   b. Levofloxacin
   c. Azithromycin
   d. Doxycycline

2. A child with fetal alcohol syndrome (FAS) is likely to exhibit which one of the following findings?
   a. Growth deficiency
   b. Normal IQ
   c. Thickened upper lip
   d. Macrocephaly

3. To evaluate a child for esotropia, which one of the following is a rapid and convenient diagnostic screening test?
   a. Slit lamp examination
   b. Corneal light reflex test
   c. Snellen test
   d. Fluorescein test

4. According to Dr. Elisabeth Kübler-Ross, dying patients experience several emotional stages during terminal illness. Which one of these emotions persists throughout all the stages of terminal illness?
   a. Anger
   b. Hope
   c. Denial
   d. Bargaining

5. You are assessing an 11-month-old African-American child who was brought in by his mother for concerns about swelling in both hands and both feet. On your examination, you find tenderness and obvious swelling of the hands and feet. Vital signs, including temperature and blood pressure, are normal. The most likely diagnosis is
   a. Osteomyelitis
   b. Hand-foot-mouth disease
   c. Glomerulonephritis
   d. Sickle cell disease

6. A 65-year-old woman complains of urinary incontinence. She is experiencing leakage of urine when she coughs, sneezes, or laughs. This form of urinary incontinence is called
    a. Stress incontinence
    b. Urge incontinence
    c. Overflow incontinence
    d. Functional incontinence

7. A full-term newborn weighed 7 pounds, 9 ounces at birth. Three days after hospital discharge, you are seeing the baby for his first checkup. He now weighs 7 pounds, 4 ounces. This level of weight loss is
    a. Worrisome because it is below birth weight
    b. Indicative of inadequate nutrition
    c. A sign of dehydration
    d. Normal at this age

8. Which of the following drugs is NOT associated with human teratogenicity?
    a. Valproic acid
    b. Warfarin
    c. Phenytoin
    d. Amoxicillin

9. An adolescent patient presents with severe sore throat, fever, cervical lymphadenopathy, and difficulty opening the mouth. On examination, you see that the uvula is deviated from the midline and there is some bulging of the soft palate near the tonsillar area. What is the most likely diagnosis?
    a. Epiglottitis
    b. Viral pharyngitis
    c. Peritonsillar abscess
    d. Retropharyngeal abscess

10. Most cases of infectious pharyngitis are caused by
    a. viruses
    b. Group A streptococcus
    c. Streptococcus pneumoniae
    d. Haemophilus influenzae

11. A pediatric patient has a tender, boggy lesion on the scalp. There are numerous pustules overlying the lesion. Occipital lymphadenopathy is also present, and there are also three to four small scaly areas of hair loss scattered over the scalp. A Wood's lamp examination shows no fluorescence. What is the most likely diagnosis?
    a. Scalp abscess
    b. Tinea capitis
    c. Impetigo
    d. MRSA infection

12. Which one of the following is a typical characteristic of *Mycoplasma pneumoniae* infection?
    a. Consolidated infiltrate on chest x-ray
    b. Headaches
    c. Hypoxia
    d. Myositis

13. Thelarche begins in girls during which Tanner stage?
    a. Stage I
    b. Stage II
    c. Stage III
    d. Stage IV

14. A nurse practitioner is examining a 55-year-old diabetic man who reports a bilateral pretibial rash. The physical exam reveals a thin epidermis with brown–yellow ulcerated plaques that are oozing blood. What is the most likely diagnosis?
    a. Erythema nodosum
    b. Myxedema
    c. Cutaneous Candida albicans infection
    d. Necrobiosis lipoidica diabeticorum (NLD)

15. Red blood cell (RBC) casts in the urine indicate
    a. interstitial nephritis
    b. myoglobinuria
    c. renal tubular damage
    d. glomerular disease

16. Which of the following is NOT a criterion for diagnosis of diabetes mellitus?
    a. Fasting blood glucose > 126 mg/dL
    b. HgA1c of 6.5%
    c. Polydipsia and polyuria
    d. Nonfasting blood glucose > 200 mg/dL

17. According to federal law, a family nurse practitioner can care for nursing home patients under which of the following conditions?
    a. A physician must be available for emergencies
    b. Patients must be younger than 80 years of age
    c. The caseload must not exceed five patients
    d. All of the above

18. An African-American woman asks a nurse practitioner about sickle cell disease. She informs the practitioner that she is homozygous for hemoglobin A (AA) and her husband has sickle cell trait (AS). What is the probability that they would have a child with sickle cell disease?
    a. 0%
    b. 25%
    c. 50%
    d. 100%

19. The percentage of persons with dementia cared for in the home by family members is closest to
    a. 33%
    b. 52%
    c. 65%
    d. 80%

20. Which of the following is a HIPAA violation?
    a. Discussing patient treatment information with another provider via e-mail
    b. Leaving patient charts outside patient exam rooms while they wait to see the provider
    c. Revealing protected health information with a pharmaceutical representative who needs feedback on his new product
    d. Releasing health information to the police to aid in an investigation

21. Which of the following is NOT a cause of secondary hypertension?
    a. Sepsis
    b. Cocaine use
    c. Kidney disease
    d. Oral contraceptive use

22. An otherwise healthy patient was diagnosed with influenza B within 48 hours of onset of symptoms and was treated with oseltamivir (Tamiflu). Within 24 hours, he reports intermittent heart palpitations. The most likely cause of the palpitations is
    a. a routine symptom of the flu virus
    b. high fever
    c. viral myocarditis
    d. a side effect of Tamiflu

23. A three-year-old-boy has had fever of 104 to 105 degrees for six days. While examining the patient, a nurse practitioner notes a strawberry tongue, a maculopapular rash on the trunk, unilateral cervical lymphadenopathy, and nonexudative conjunctivitis. He also has cracked lips and edema of the hands and feet. A physician treated the patient three days prior with antibiotics for a presumed strep infection. What is the most likely diagnosis?
    a. Toxic epidermal necrolysis
    b. Resistant strep infection
    c. Kawasaki disease
    d. Juvenile rheumatoid arthritis

24. An American elderly person is most likely to be abused by which one of the following?
    a. A sibling
    b. A spouse
    c. A daughter
    d. An unrelated caregiver

25. Which one of these conditions is associated with the highest suicide rate?
    a. COPD
    b. Diabetes
    c. AIDS
    d. Osteoporosis

26. The most common cause of viral pneumonia in adults is
    a. adenovirus
    b. RSV
    c. Haemophilus influenzae
    d. influenza virus

27. A family nurse practitioner is evaluating a 21-year-old patient with bilateral eye irritation. He has had several similar episodes in the past, but this one is more severe. The palpebral conjunctivae are edematous and velvety red and the bulbar conjunctivae are injected. No eye discharge is visible. Which one of these other clinical findings would you expect to see in this case?
    a. Increased intraocular pressure
    b. Fever
    c. Myopia
    d. Pruritus

28. All of the following are nonsteroidal anti-inflammatory drugs EXCEPT
    a. acetylsalicylic acid
    b. acetaminophen
    c. indomethacin
    d. naproxen

29. The most common cause of cancer-related deaths in the 25- to 44-year-olds group is
    a. lung cancer
    b. Hodgkin's lymphoma
    c. breast cancer
    d. colon cancer

30. An adult patient with iron deficiency anemia asks you about foods that are rich in iron. Which one of the following is highest in iron?
    a. Oranges
    b. Whole milk
    c. Beans
    d. Egg whites

31. A 21-month old child has a fever of 103 degrees, fussiness, drooling, and lack of appetite. On exam, you note a red throat with several ulcerations over the tonsillar pillars. What is the most likely diagnosis?
    a. Herpangina
    b. Strep pharyngitis
    c. Gingivostomatitis
    d. Epiglottitis

32. Which of the following is not an etiologic agent of bronchiolitis?
    a. RSV
    b. Coronavirus
    c. Norovirus
    d. Rhinovirus

33. A family nurse practitioner has a patient who is habitually at least 30 minutes late for her appointments. She is a 42-year-old Hispanic woman with several health issues. Which of the following statements demonstrates cultural competence on the part of the healthcare provider?
    a. The provider should not take cultural differences into account in healthcare situations
    b. Refusing to see the patient unless she arrives on time will teach her a lesson
    c. Consider that the patient belongs to a culture where being on time is flexible or approximate rather than exact
    d. Making a reminder call to the patient the day before will solve the problem

34. Pneumococcal polysaccharide vaccine (PPSV 23, Pneumovax) is
    a. recommended for all adults age 65 or over
    b. administered intradermally
    c. recommended yearly for asplenic patients
    d. not given concurrently with other vaccines

35. The number-one cause of blindness in the elderly is
    a. cataracts
    b. age-related macular degeneration
    c. glaucoma
    d. diabetic retinopathy

36. A family nurse practitioner is evaluating a three-year-old child with suspected Henoch–Schönlein purpura (HSP). Which one of the following is NOT true about HSP?
    a. Patients may complain of joint pain
    b. The purpura is due thrombocytopenia
    c. HSP may be associated with abdominal pain
    d. Microscopic hematuria may be present

37. Which one of the following is good advice for a patient with gastroesophageal reflux disease (GERD)?
    a. Take anticholinergics to speed gastric emptying
    b. Increase fat intake
    c. Raise the head of the bed on two-inch blocks
    d. Eat a high-fiber diet

38. A family nurse practitioner is instructing a 65-year-old patient on taking psyllium (Metamucil). Which of the following is appropriate advice?
    a. Sprinkle psyllium into a half cup of applesauce, and eat the entire serving
    b. Take the psyllium dose mixed in one cup of fluid followed by a second glass of fluid
    c. Psyllium is most effective when taken with a calcium supplement
    d. The onset of action of psyllium is usually within 30 to 45 minutes

39. What is the treatment of choice for a routine tooth abscess?
    a. Extraction of the tooth
    b. Erythromycin
    c. Penicillin VK
    d. Levaquin

40. A nurse practitioner is seeing an adult patient with a 72-hour history of fever, cough, and runny nose. Her in-clinic flu test is positive for flu type B. She wants a prescription for antibiotics. Which one of the following would be the best thing to tell her?
    a. "The virus will just have to run its course. Be patient."
    b. "There's just nothing I can do to cure a virus."
    c. "Everybody knows antibiotics are not effective for treating the flu."
    d. "You must feel miserable and I sympathize with you. Let's discuss some things that will relieve your symptoms."

41. Which of the following statements is true about an infantile umbilical hernia?
    a. It will most likely require surgical repair
    b. It will get worse if the baby cries excessively
    c. The baby should wear a band around the abdomen to keep the hernia "in"
    d. It will heal on its own because it is less than 2 cm in diameter

42. The family members of a patient with Alzheimer's disease are having difficulty coping with the patient's repetition of questions and phrases. This phenomenon is known as
    a. perseveration
    b. denial
    c. confabulation
    d. contrivance

43. A nurse practitioner instructing a newly diagnosed diabetic on the symptoms of hypoglycemia. Which one of the following is NOT a symptom of hypoglycemia?
    a. diaphoresis
    b. tremors
    c. hunger
    d. diplopia

44. Which of these choices best describes the classic presentation of viral croup in a toddler?
    a. Drooling and sitting in a tripod position
    b. Seal-like cough and rhinorrhea
    c. Fever of 104.5 and cough
    d. Oxygen saturation of 92% and severe retractions

45. A nurse practitioner is performing a breast exam on a 44-year-old woman and detects a painless irregular-shaped mass on the right breast. Which one of these findings is most likely to be associated with breast cancer?
    a. Breast lump fixed to muscle or skin
    b. A tender nodule
    c. Nodule that feels rubbery
    d. Lumps in both breasts

46. The mechanism of injury in a nursemaid's elbow is usually
    a. pulling
    b. twisting
    c. bending
    d. compression

47. A family nurse practitioner is conducting a follow-up visit with a 60-year-old woman who is on Coumadin for a history of deep vein thrombosis originally treated in the hospital. She is in the clinic today for an exam and to have her INR checked. The goal for her INR is
    a. 1.2
    b. 2 to 3
    c. 4.0
    d. 4 to 4.5

48. A 42-year-old man wants to quit smoking. He wants to know the symptoms of nicotine withdrawal. All of the following are symptoms EXCEPT
    a. difficulty sleeping
    b. tachycardia
    c. anxiety
    d. impotence

49. A mother brings her nine-month-old son to see the nurse practitioner for a tight foreskin. What is the best management approach?
    a. Force the foreskin back under direct physician supervision
    b. Refer the baby to a urologist
    c. Advise the mother to retract the foreskin little by little at each diaper change until it loosens
    d. Explain to the mother that a tight foreskin is normal at this age

50. Which one of the following is a conjugated vaccine?
    a. Inactivated polio vaccine
    b. Hepatitis B vaccine
    c. Hib vaccine
    d. Acellular pertussis vaccine

51. The rotavirus vaccine is given to children to protect against a potentially severe diarrheal infection. An early version of the vaccine was removed from the market because of its association with
    a. a high risk of developing the rotavirus infection after vaccination
    b. a contaminant in the vaccine
    c. an increased risk of intussusception
    d. poor development of immunity after vaccination

52. A family nurse practitioner has given an influenza vaccine to an adult patient. The patient wants to know how long it will take for his body to form antibodies to the virus. Your answer is
    a. 4 to 6 weeks
    b. 72 hours
    c. 48 hours
    d. 2 weeks

53. Due to visual impairment and problems with mobility, an elderly patient is unable to care for himself. In reference to barriers against self-care, these two specific impairments are classified as
    a. cognitive barriers
    b. physical barriers
    c. psychological barriers
    d. psychosocial barriers

54. Which of these is NOT associated with infant tooth decay?
    a. Exclusive breastfeeding
    b. Sleeping with a bottle of formula in the mouth
    c. Frequent pacifier use
    d. Presence of only one to four erupted teeth

55. At what age(s) can one begin to obtain reliable hearing screening results?
    a. Newborn
    b. Age six months
    c. Age nine months
    d. Ages two to three years

56. Which of the following is true about eye contact in the clinical setting?
    a. Eye contact occurs in generally the same way from one culture to another
    b. In some cultures, direct eye contact is considered to be rude
    c. In American culture, avoiding eye contact is usually a signal of respect for the other person
    d. Avoiding direct eye contact is always a sign of disapproval

57. Which statement correctly pertains to delegation of tasks to unlicensed assistants?
    a. It is unnecessary for the nurse practitioner to provide general instructions for the task
    b. Once the task is clearly explained, the nurse practitioner need not provide ongoing supervision
    c. If the assistant needs help with the task, she can get help from another unlicensed assistant who is unfamiliar with the task
    d. The delegating nurse practitioner is ultimately accountable for completion of the task

58. Which of the following is an example of medical negligence?
    a. Delegating a routine task to a trained assistant
    b. Failure to monitor a patient
    c. Providing medical advice over the phone
    d. Referring a patient to a specialist

59. Which of these statements is true about the nurse practitioner scope of practice?
    a. Nurse practitioners may not prescribe narcotics in most states
    b. Nurse practitioner scopes of practice vary widely from state to state
    c. Most states allow nurse practitioners to practice independently
    d. A nurse practitioner cannot evaluate the psychosocial status of a patient

60. Scabies is an infestation caused by
    a. Mites
    b. Insects
    c. Ticks
    d. Protozoans

61. Which of these is NOT a potential complication of rosacea?
    a. Folliculitis
    b. Oral lesions
    c. Facial pyoderma
    d. Dry eyes

62. A possible complication of gallstones is
    a. hepatitis
    b. gastritis
    c. acute cholecystitis
    d. cancer of the gallbladder

63. Which of the following is the most appropriate treatment for a single tinea corporis lesion that is less than 2 cm in diameter?
    a. Topical betamethasone
    b. Oral griseofulvin
    c. Topical diphenhydramine
    d. Topical clotrimazole

64. The percentage of patients with Bell's palsy that experience full and spontaneous resolution is closest to
    a. 25%
    b. 50%
    c. 70%
    d. 90%

65. A key component in the initial overall management of osteoarthritis is
    a. nonpharmacologic treatment
    b. etanercept (Enbrel)
    c. joint replacement surgery
    d. arthroscopy

66. Management of a 34-year-old man with Type 2 diabetes routinely includes all of these EXCEPT
    a. referral to an ophthalmologist for periodic retinal exams
    b. measuring lipid levels periodically
    c. screen for proteinuria periodically
    d. measuring HbA1c once yearly

67. A nurse practitioner is assessing a "suspicious" mole on a 78-year-old man's face. He is concerned about skin cancer. The most common type of skin cancer is
    a. squamous cell carcinoma
    b. melanoma
    c basal cell carcinoma
    d. mycosis fungoides

68. A nurse practitioner is performing a Denver II Developmental Screening Test on a toddler. Which of the following is NOT a developmental category screened by the test?
    a. Fine motor development
    b. Language development
    c. Gross motor development
    d. Emotional development

69. A nurse practitioner is counseling a pregnant woman about the risks of smoking during pregnancy. Which one of the following is associated with smoking during pregnancy?
    a. Gestational diabetes
    b. Preeclampsia
    c. Low birth weight
    d. Molar pregnancy

70. Which of the following has a protective effect against the development of neural tube defects during pregnancy?
    a. Vitamin B12
    b. Iron sulfate
    c. Folic acid
    d. Vitamin C

71. The mother of a nine-year-old girl is concerned that the child is already showing signs of breast development. What would you do next?
    a. Reassure the mother that breast development at this age is within normal limits
    b. Make a diagnosis of premature breast development
    c. Refer the child to an endocrinologist
    d. Obtain bone age radiographs

72. During a routine physical exam, a family nurse practitioner notices peripheral edema of both legs in a 48-year-old diabetic woman who also suffers from high blood pressure and depression. Of the following medications, which of the following is most likely causing the edema?
    a. Hydrochlorothiazide
    b. Fluoxetine (Prozac)
    c. Rosiglitazone (Avandia)
    d. Metformin

73. In general, all of the following should have a preoperative electrocardiogram EXCEPT
    a. men over age 45
    b. patients with known heart disease
    c. patients with a history of costochondritis
    d. patients with hypertension

74. At what age would it be appropriate to stop performing Pap smears on a 53-year-old woman whose previous Pap smears have all been normal? Both she and her husband have been monogamous for 30 years.

    a. 60 years

    b. 65 years

    c. 70 years

    d. She should continue Pap screenings indefinitely

75. A 66-year-old woman with asthma states she has not received any immunizations since age 14 years. Aside from her asthma, she is healthy. She asks you if she currently needs any vaccines. Which one of the following would you recommend?

    a. FluMist

    b. Pneumovax

    c. MMR

    d. Hib

76. You have diagnosed a 32-year-old woman with influenza A. She wants prophylaxis with oseltamivir (Tamiflu) for her two children, ages 2 months and 2 years. Which of these choices represents the current influenza prophylaxis recommendations?

    a. Only the 2 month old may receive prophylaxis

    b. Only the 4 year old may receive prophylaxis

    c. Both may receive prophylaxis

    d. Neither may receive prophylaxis

77. In reference to patient education, which one of these statements is true?

    a. Patients usually recall and understand most information given by their provider

    b. Most patients feel their providers overload them with information

    c. When behavioral changes are medically necessary, patients like to be given options for change and then select from the list

    d. Leaning toward the patient while giving instructions does not increase recall

78. A family nurse practitioner is working in a clinic that sees many Native-American patients. Which of these health conditions has a higher prevalence among Native Americans when compared to other American population groups?

    a. Tuberculosis

    b. Hypertension

    c. Coronary artery disease

    d. Obesity

79. Which one of the following is NOT one of the three fundamental principles of professionalism?

    a. Principle of professional appearance

    b. Primacy of patient welfare

    c. Principle of patient autonomy

    d. Principle of social justice

80. A 42-year-old man has terminal cancer. He will most likely die within one year. He asks you not to disclose this prognosis to his wife. You see his wife as you are walking out of the hospital and she asks you to "tell her the truth" about her husband's condition. You feel she has a right to know, and you tell her about the grim prognosis. This is a violation of
    a. Patient autonomy
    b. Patient welfare
    c. Patient confidentiality
    d. Professional competence

81. Which of the following is NOT an area of concern when giving parents anticipatory guidance for a two-year-old?
    a. Physical development
    b. Emotional development
    c. Sexual development
    d. Safety issues

82. A 46-year-old man presents for evaluation of a red rash on both cheeks. This is his third flare-up of the same problem. Some red papules and pustules are visible in the involved areas. On closer inspection, you notice some telangiectasias on his nose and cheeks. There are no comedones present. What is the most likely diagnosis?
    a. Lupus erythematosus
    b. Acne
    c. Rosacea
    d. Seborrheic dermatitis

83. A patient was diagnosed with right temporomandibular joint dysfunction several months ago. She now presents for evaluation of right ear pain. The most likely etiology of her ear pain is
    a. Eustachian tube dysfunction
    b. otitis media
    c. otitis externa
    d. referred pain

84. Which of these conditions most commonly predisposes a patient to recurrent bacterial sinusitis?
    a. Immune system deficiency
    b. Allergic rhinitis
    c. GERD
    d. Cigarette smoking

85. A family nurse practitioner is discussing a treatment plan with an adult patient. The patient is sitting with arms folded across his chest, his legs crossed at the knees, and he is leaning backward. Which type of nonverbal communication is he exhibiting?
    a. Body language
    b. Gestures
    c. Facial expressions
    d. Empathy

86. A family nurse practitioner is caring for a patient who speaks only Vietnamese. A Vietnamese interpreter is present to help. Which of these statements best describes appropriate behavior when using an interpreter?
  a. Express two to three ideas at a time before pausing for the interpreter to speak to the patient
  b. Speak clearly and loudly
  c. Face the interpreter when you speak
  d. If the patient gives an unusual response to a question, ask your question in a different way

87. A physician has asked a nurse practitioner to give discharge instructions to a patient. The nurse practitioner notices that the physician has prescribed amoxicillin to a patient with a documented penicillin allergy. What is the appropriate action for the nurse practitioner to take?
  a. No action is needed because penicillin and amoxicillin belong to different families of drugs
  b. Assume that the physician knows best and keep quiet
  c. Call the error to the physician's attention in a professional manner
  d. Tell the patient that the physician is incompetent

88. Which of the following is a "red flag" for patient drug-seeking behavior?
  a. The patient claims allergies to multiple classes of non-narcotic pain medications
  b. The patient is using relaxation techniques under medical supervision for relief of pain
  c. The patient has tried acupuncture
  d. The patient becomes upset when not treated with antibiotics for a virus

89. An adult female with a vaginal discharge presents for evaluation. You order a KOH prep on the discharge. The laboratory reports the presence of clue cells. The best treatment for this patient is
  a. doxycycline
  b. ceftriaxone
  c. terconazole
  d. metronidazole

90. Fifth disease is caused by
  a. a parvovirus
  b. an enterovirus
  c. a paramyxovirus
  d. an adenovirus

91. Which one of the following medications is clearly contraindicated during pregnancy?
  a. Amoxicillin
  b. Ondansetron (Zofran)
  c. Permethrin 5% cream (Elimite)
  d. Isotretinoin (Accutane)

92. The problem-solving process has various components. When identifying a problem, a family nurse practitioner employs the nursing process of
    a. planning
    b. assessment
    c. implementation
    d. evaluation

93. If two nurse practitioners have incompatible differences in values and patient care beliefs, which type of conflict exists between them?
    a. Organizational
    b. Intrapersonal
    c. Interpersonal
    d. Psychological

94. A nurse needs rehabilitation for addiction to narcotics and is now unable to function in her profession. She has agreed to attend Narcotics Anonymous, file a quarterly report with the board of nursing, work daytime hours, and work in a nursing unit where narcotics are not available. What term best describes this situation?
    a. Diversion program
    b. Public reprimand
    c. Probation
    d. Licensure revocation

95. When two or more states recognize licensure by other state boards that have equivalent licensing requirements, this is known as
    a. temporary license
    b. licensing by waiver
    c. licensure by examination
    d. reciprocity

96. Before delegating a task to unlicensed assistive personnel, the nurse must check that all of the following exist EXCEPT
    a. low risk of harm to the patient
    b. adequate opportunity for supervision
    c. delegation of a complex problem-solving task
    d. highly predictable task outcome

97. All of the following are categories of medication errors EXCEPT
    a. wrong patient
    b. incorrect dosage
    c. failure to note patient allergies
    d. surgical removal of wrong body part

98. A nurse feels that a physician's error may cause harm to a patient. In order to ensure patient safety, she disobeys the order and notifies a nursing supervisor. Under this circumstance, the nurse is acting as a
    a. whistleblower
    b. patient advocate
    c. nursing advocate
    d. legal advisor

99. A process that analyzes, identifies, and treats potential hazards in a specific setting is known as
   a. risk management
   b. quality assurance
   c. standards of care
   d. patient rights

100. A nurse discovers a patient lying on the floor of his hospital room but did not actually see what happened. She initiates an incident report. Which of the following is the best way to document the incident?
   a. The patient most likely slipped on a wet spot on the floor
   b. The patient apparently fainted and fell to the floor
   c. The patient was going to the bathroom, lost his balance, and fell down
   d. The patient was found lying face-down on the floor of his room

101. Nurse practice acts
   a. are statutes established by state legislatures to regulate nursing practice in each state
   b. do not define the scope of nursing practice
   c. establish policies for prevention and resolution of ethical dilemmas
   d. are the same for every state

102. A nurse working in a hospital setting is frustrated and overwhelmed with work because of inadequate staffing. She is considering walking out and leaving the hospital. If she leaves, she could be charged with
   a. fraud
   b. defamation
   c. abandonment
   d. collective bargaining

103. All of the following are true about incident reports EXCEPT
   a. Incident reports can be useful in improving patient care and in identifying risks
   b. Incident reports should be completed accurately
   c. The report form should be copied and placed in the patient record
   d. The report should be filled out following specific documentation guidelines

104. A 25-year-old patient is having trouble with recurrent conjunctivitis, having had four episodes in the past year. She wears contact lenses. What type of organisms should be strongly suspected as a cause of eye infections in contact lens wearers?
   a. Gram-negative organisms
   b. Fungi
   c. Adenoviruses
   d. Mixed organisms

105. You are evaluating an eight-month-old child whose mother reports a history of frequent vomiting over the past two months. She has mentioned it to other providers, but she has been told the baby would "outgrow it." In looking over his medical record, you notice the patient has also been seen for recurrent episodes of wheezing. However, he is currently not wheezing, is afebrile, and appears healthy. Which of the following is the most likely cause of the vomiting?

    a. Pyloric stenosis
    b. Gastroesophageal reflux (GER)
    c. Gastroenteritis
    d. Reactive airway disease

106. A 30-year-old woman has a body mass index (BMI) of 28. According to her BMI, the patient is

    a. normal weight
    b. overweight
    c. obese
    d. extremely obese

107. The percentage of Americans that are overweight (based on BMI) is closest to

    a. 20%
    b. 35%
    c. 50%
    d. 65%

108. A four-year-old child presents with a complaint of rust-colored urine. She has no dysuria and no history of urinary tract infections in the past. She has been healthy except for a recent case of impetigo, which has since resolved. Her mother states that the child's eyes looked "a little puffy" this morning, but look fine now. Which of the following is the most likely diagnosis?

    a. UTI
    b. Kidney stone
    c. Poststreptococcal glomerulonephritis
    d. Nephrotic syndrome

109. An adult patient with persistent sinusitis has failed treatment with amoxicillin, trimethoprim/sulfa, and amoxicillin clavulanate. Which of the following is the best choice for the next round of treatment?

    a. A first-generation cephalosporin
    b. Clarithromycin
    c. A fluoroquinolone
    d. Erythromycin ethylsuccinate

110. A 38-year-old man developed lower back pain that started two days after lifting up his four-year-old son. He has limited spinal range of motion, but his neurological exam is normal. You suspect nerve root irritation from a herniated disk. Which of the following would help corroborate the diagnosis?

    a. An MRI
    b. Plain lumbosacral radiographs
    c. Testing range of spinal motion
    d. Bend-over test

111. You are discussing avoidance of asthma triggers with an adult patient. Which of these offers the best advice?
   a. Vacuum carpets daily to remove allergens
   b. Use ceiling fans throughout the home instead of air conditioning
   c. Maintain home humidity levels over 50%
   d. Encase his mattress and pillows in allergen-blocking covers

112. Which of these antidepressants is least likely to cause sexual side effects?
   a. Bupropion (Wellbutrin)
   b. Escitalopram (Lexapro)
   c. Amitriptyline (Elavil)
   d. Fluoxetine (Prozac)

113. A 55-year-old woman has swelling of the proximal interphalangeal joints of the first and second digits of both hands. She also complains of prolonged morning stiffness and often experiences excessive fatigue. What is the most likely diagnosis?
   a. Gout
   b. Osteoarthritis
   c. Rheumatoid arthritis
   d. Psoriatic arthritis

114. A 64-year-old man presents with acute onset of redness and severe pain in his right eye. He also complains of blurred vision, headache, nausea, and seeing halos around lights. After examining the patient and taking a history, what is your next course of action?
   a. Reassure the patient and prescribe antibiotic eye drops for conjunctivitis
   b. Apply tetracaine drops to relieve pain
   c. Perform a fluorescein test to check for a corneal abrasion
   d. Arrange for immediate referral to an ophthalmologist

115. A 6-month-old infant has been diagnosed and hospitalized with pertussis. The infant is not in daycare. The only known sick contact is a 12-year-old sibling who has had a cough for 3 weeks. Which of the following represents the best option for chemoprophylaxis in this case?
   a. Treat all household contacts and other close contacts with erythromycin
   b. Treat only the sibling who has the cough and the sick infant
   c. Treat all household and other close contacts with either azithromycin or clarithromycin
   d. If all other close contacts are current on their immunizations, there is no need for prophylaxis

116. A nine-month-old Caucasian child has been seen in your clinic for frequent respiratory infections and frequent bouts with loose stools. Stool cultures and ova and parasites have been negative. During her routine physical examination, you discover that in the past four months her growth parameters have dropped from the 60th percentile to the 10th percentile for weight and from the 75th percentile to the 25th percentile for height. What is the best thing to do next?
   a. Order thyroid function tests
   b. Order a sweat chloride test
   c. Admit the child to the hospital to see if she gains weight when fed appropriately
   d. Evaluate for tuberculosis

117. You are evaluating a newborn infant for a Moro reflex. Of the following, which is the best way to elicit the reflex?
    a. Gently stroke the perioral area with a finger
    b. Turn the newborn's head to one side, and observe his arm movements
    c. Apply firm pressure to the palm of the baby's hand
    d. Clap your hands loudly and suddenly

118. Which of the following is useful as a rescue medication in the treatment of asthma?
    a. Corticosteroid inhaler
    b. Leukotriene inhibitor
    c. Anti-allergic medications
    d. Short-acting beta-2 agonist

119. Which of the following is most likely to be the first symptom of tuberculosis?
    a. Chest pain
    b. Cough productive of bloody sputum
    c. Mild cough with nonbloody mucoid sputum
    d. Shortness of breath

120. An 11-month-old baby recently completed a course of oral antibiotics for otitis media. She now presents with a beefy red rash in the diaper area. The rash is surrounded by small satellite lesions and has not responded to diaper rash ointments. What is the best way to manage this rash?
    a. Prescribe topical nystatin cream
    b. Advise the parents to apply talcum powder at each diaper change
    c. Prescribe mupirocin ointment
    d. Prescribe oral fluconazole

121. A 10-year-old girl has a two-week history of a mucocele inside her lower lip. There is no pain or bleeding. What is your next course of action?
    a. Manually rupture the lesion and let the contents flow out
    b. Cauterize the lesion with silver nitrate
    c. Advise the parents that spontaneous rupture will occur
    d. Refer immediately to an oral surgeon

122. Which one of the following is true about primary enuresis in children?
    a. A physical etiology, such as a UTI, is found in about 20% of children
    b. Bed wetting is more common in boys than girls
    c. The patient should take imipramine
    d. It is crucial to perform a renal ultrasound as soon as possible

123. A four-year-old child presents with a four-day history of cough and nasal congestion. He had a temperature of 100.8 for the initial 24 hours only. Today, his nasal mucus is thicker and yellow. What is the most likely diagnosis?
    a. Allergic rhinitis
    b. Sinusitis
    c. Viral upper respiratory infection (URI)
    d. Foreign body in the nose

124. A 21-year-old asymptomatic woman has a positive purified protein derivative (PPD) test result of 13 mm. What is the next step in managing this patient?
   a. Chest x-ray
   b. Chest x-ray and six to nine months of treatment with isoniazid (INH)
   c. Sputum culture
   d. Repeat the PPD in three months

125. Which of the following patients is at increased risk for recurrent otitis media?
   a. A teenager on the school swimming team
   b. A child with narrow ear canals
   c. A child with cleft palate
   d. An infant with blocked tear ducts

126. All of the following are associated with childhood exposure to cigarette smoke EXCEPT
   a. Colic
   b. Bacterial conjunctivitis
   c. SIDS
   d. Wheezing

127. Which of these illnesses is most frequently reported by patients who have recently traveled overseas?
   a. Hepatitis A
   b. Traveler's diarrhea
   c. Malaria
   d. Amoebiasis

128. Which of the following types of patients is most likely to be interested in using alternative medical therapies?
   a. Patients older than age 65
   b. Men
   c. Women
   d. High school and college students

129. A two-year old child has viral diarrhea. Several other children in his daycare have the same illness. He is not vomiting and is eating well. His mother asks for treatment recommendations. What would you do next?
   a. Advise his mother to keep the child well hydrated
   b. Recommend Imodium AD
   c. Prescribe Levsin
   d. Tell the mother to stop solid foods for now

130. A 72-year-old man complains of cramping pain in both calves after walking. The pain disappears after resting. His condition is most likely
   a. restless legs syndrome
   b. multiple sclerosis
   c. intermittent claudication
   d. normal for his age

131. Which one of the following about the erythrocyte sedimentation rate (ESR) is true?
   a. It measures the rate red blood cells fall in an upright tube of anticoagulated blood in a 30-minute period
   b. It is a specific test for inflammation
   c. It is an acute phase reactant
   d. The faster the red blood cells fall, the higher the sedimentation rate

132. A young and inexperienced mother brings in her 6-month-old infant for evaluation of vomiting and diarrhea. Because he has been vomiting his formula, the baby's mother has been giving him nothing but plain water for the past 24 hours. The infant suddenly has a seizure in the clinic. Of the following choices, he is most likely suffering from
   a. hyponatremia
   b. sepsis
   c. idiopathic epilepsy
   d. carotenemia

133. The Adams forward bend test is used to
   a. screen for scoliosis
   b. test for a herniated disk
   c. assess cerebellar function
   d. assess for spinal arthritis

134. Contributory negligence occurs when
   a. the healthcare provider willfully disregards the safety of the patient
   b. the healthcare provider fails to provide appropriate standard of care
   c. the patient contributes to his own negative outcome
   d. a percentage of negligence is assigned to each party involved

135. A patient weighs 64 kilograms and is 1.6 meters tall. What is her body mass index (BMI)?
   a. 22
   b. 25
   c. 28
   d. 30

136. A mother tells you that her two-year-old child refuses almost all solid foods. She states, "All he'll take is whole milk." This child is most at risk for
   a. hemolytic anemia
   b. developing milk allergy
   c. gastroesophageal reflux
   d. iron deficiency anemia

137. A 79-year-old multiparous woman complains of a pulling sensation in her vagina and bloody spotting on her underwear. She has also started to have some mild urinary incontinence. As you prepare to examine the area, you notice a rather large ulcerated soft tissue mass at the vaginal introitus. What is the most likely diagnosis?
   a. Urethral prolapse
   b. Uterine prolapse
   c. Vaginal neoplasm
   d. Pelvic hernia

138. Which of the following is NOT a symptom of retinal detachment?
   a. Eye pain
   b. Flashes of light
   c. Floaters
   d. Loss of central vision

139. Which of the following hernias is most likely to be acquired?
   a. Indirect inguinal hernia
   b. Direct inguinal hernia
   c. Infant umbilical hernia
   d. Hiatal hernia in a child

140. An elderly, immobile patient in a nursing home has a well-defined area of nontender persistent redness in the sacral area. The skin is still intact. What is the most likely explanation for this condition?
   a. Cellulitis
   b. Abscess
   c. Stage 1 bedsore
   d. Ant bite

141. All of the following are grounds for nursing malpractice EXCEPT
   a. failure to report a change in a patient's condition
   b. neglecting to monitor a patient properly
   c. administering a medication not ordered by the physician
   d. failure to maintain continuing education requirements

142. An adolescent complains of acute left ear pain. The ear hurts with manipulation of the external ear. On examination, the ear canal is red, swollen, and very tender. You also notice flaky debris in the ear canal. Which of the following is the most appropriate treatment?
   a. Antipyrine/benzocaine ear drops (Auralgan)
   b. Combination antibiotic and corticosteroid ear drops
   c. Ibuprofen and warm compresses to the ear
   d. Oral antibiotics

143. You are performing a developmental exam on a child. He is able to use a pincer grasp, pull up to stand, and he understands the word "no." His age is closest to
   a. 4 months
   b. 5 months
   c. 6 months
   d. 9 months

144. An obviously distressed 14-year-old boy has recently noticed that one of his breasts has grown larger than the other and is also somewhat tender. His mother seems equally concerned. What is the best management course to follow?
   a. Treat for mastitis
   b. Offer reassurance that this is temporary and benign
   c. Check testosterone levels
   d. Refer him to an endocrinologist

145. Which of the following is the best way to stop a nosebleed?
    a. Apply an ice pack to the forehead
    b. Apply pressure on the bridge of the nose
    c. Pinch nostrils shut and apply pressure for 10 continuous minutes
    d. Have the patient relax and tilt his head back

146. An 81-year-old woman complains of darkening of the skin right above her ankles, itching, thinning of the skin, and progressive irritation. Her ankles swell intermittently. What is the most likely diagnosis?
    a. Venous stasis dermatitis
    b. Zinc deficiency
    c. Atopic dermatitis
    d. Id reaction

147. A known asthmatic has a peak flow meter reading that is 78% of his personal best. This measurement is in the
    a. normal zone
    b. green zone
    c. yellow zone
    d. red zone

148. In reference to adult CPR, the currently recommended ratio of chest compressions to breaths is
    a. 15:2
    b. 10:2
    c. dependent on the age of the patient
    d. 30:2

149. Which of the following is the best prophylactic treatment for traveler's diarrhea in an adult?
    a. Amoxicillin
    b. Ciprofloxacin
    c. Trimethoprim/sulfa
    d. Doxycycline

150. Which of the following is the treatment of choice for an adult female with gonococcal cervicitis?
    a. Penicillin intramuscularly
    b. Ceftriaxone intramuscularly
    c. Oral doxycycline for seven days
    d. Oral azithromycin

Answers and Explanations

1. C: Only azithromycin has shown effectiveness when taken as a single dose for treatment of chlamydial urethritis. Levofloxacin and doxycycline are also effective treatment choices, but would have to be taken for seven days. Ceftriaxone (Rocephin) is not effective in this case.

2. A: FAS is caused by alcohol consumption during pregnancy. Pregnant women should be counseled against drinking any amount of alcohol because there is no known "safe" amount to
drink. Pregnant women should abstain from alcohol during all trimesters. Alcohol has a wide range of permanent effects on children, particularly on the nervous system. Some common characteristics include abnormal facial features (thin upper lip and smooth philtrum), microcephaly, growth deficiency, hyperactivity, learning disabilities, and low IQ.

3. B: Corneal reflex tests are useful to diagnose strabismus. To perform the test, shine a light directly onto both corneas at the same time with the patient looking straight at the light source. In patients with strabismus (e.g., esotropia), the light reflected on the cornea appears off-center in the affected eye. Note that corneal light reflex tests may not detect an intermittent strabismus.

4. B: The five emotional stages of dying are hope, denial, isolation, anger, and bargaining. The hope of a cure (even if slim) persists throughout all the other stages of terminal illness. Isolation and denial help handle the shock of approaching death. After this, the patient experiences anger followed by bargaining.

5. D: Dactylitis (hand-foot syndrome) is often the first manifestation of sickle cell disease in an infant or toddler. Swelling and pain are usually symmetric and result from ischemia of small bones. Bone marrow is expanding and compromising circulation to the bones of the hands and feet. X rays are not helpful in the acute phase, but they eventually show bone destruction and repair. Management includes hydration and pain control. Patients who present with dactylitis before 24 months of age often go on to have a severe course of sickle cell disease.

6. A: Stress incontinence refers to leakage of urine by performance of an activity that puts pressure on the bladder. These activities include laughing, sneezing, lifting something heavy, or coughing. Urge incontinence is present when a patient develops a sudden, strong urge to urinate and begins passing urine before making it to the bathroom. Patients who have functional incontinence have a physical or mental disability that prevents normal urination even though the urinary tract is normal. Examples are Parkinson's disease, dementia, and severe depression.

7. D: Most babies lose several ounces during the first week of life. They usually get back to birth weight and start gaining weight by two weeks of age. Breastfed babies may take a little longer to get back to birth weight. A weight loss of between 5% and 10% in the first week is within normal range.

8. D: Valproic acid (Depakene, Depakote) is an anticonvulsant associated with an elevated risk of neural tube defects, such as spina bifida and meningocele, among others. Phenytoin (Dilantin) affects the developing fetus and may cause such defects as cleft lip, cleft palate, mental deficiency, and hypoplastic fingers and nails. Warfarin (Coumadin), a common anticoagulant, is known to cause nasal deformities, brain abnormalities, and stillbirth. Of the answer choices given for this question, only amoxicillin is not known as a teratogen.

9. C: Peritonsillar abscesses are typical in teens. Symptoms include sore throat, fever, and difficulty swallowing and opening the mouth (trismus). In fact, the exam may be difficult due to trismus. The abscess causes bulging of the soft palate in the tonsillar area. Cultures usually grow group A strep and mixed anaerobes. Retropharyngeal abscesses occur most frequently in children under five years of age and are less common in older patients whose retropharyngeal nodes have involuted. Epiglottitis also causes sore throat and fever, but it is accompanied by respiratory distress and typically occurs in younger children.

10. A: Viruses cause over 62% of infectious pharyngitis. The remaining answer choices are bacterial agents. Contrary to what patients often believe, group A strep pharyngitis is significantly less common than viral pharyngitis.

11. B: This patient has tinea capitis. The boggy lesion on the scalp is a kerion, which is often mistaken for an abscess. Itchy, scaly areas on the scalp and scattered areas of hair loss are common, as are swollen occipital lymph nodes. Most cases of tinea capitis in the United States are caused by *Trichophyton tonsurans,* which does not fluoresce on Wood's lamp examination. While impetigo can occur on the scalp, it is not associated with hair loss. All clinical information provided in this clinical scenario points to tinea capitis, making all other choices incorrect.

12. B: Constitutional symptoms such as malaise and headaches are typical with *Mycoplasma* infection. The expected norm for chest x-ray findings is diffuse infiltrates as opposed to a consolidated infiltrate. Myalgias and myositis are more common with viral pneumonia. Hypoxia is also atypical for pneumonia due to *Mycoplasma.*

13. B: Breast bud development (thelarche) starts during Tanner stage II. Stage I represents preadolescent girls who have not yet developed secondary sex characteristics. Stages III and IV are more advanced stages of sexual development. Stage V is the highest level of sexual development and is equivalent to an adult in sexual characteristics.

14. D: NLD is characterized by collagen degeneration, granulomatous reaction, fat deposits, and thickened blood vessel walls. The specific cause is unknown, but several theories hint at peripheral blood vessel disease, vasculitis, or trauma. Erythema nodosum usually also occurs on the pretibial areas, but consists of tender red subcutaneous nodules. Myxedema is a nonpitting edema associated with hypothyroidism. Candida infections most commonly occur in warm, moist skin folds.

15. D: Urinary casts may be composed of red blood cells, white blood cells, or renal cells. To perform a test for casts, the patient provides a midstream clean-catch urine specimen. RBC casts indicate bleeding into the renal tubule, commonly seen in glomerular diseases such as lupus nephritis, IgA nephropathy, and Wegener's granulomatosis. With renal tubular damage, renal tubular epithelial cell casts are present in the urine. Neither UTIs nor interstitial nephritis is associated with RBC casts.

16. B: Answer choices A, C, and D are all criteria for diagnosing diabetes. HgA1c is useful for periodic assessment of average glucose levels. It is not recommended for diagnostic purposes.

17. A: A nurse practitioner can care for nursing home patients as long as a physician is available in case of emergency. The restrictions mentioned in the other answer choices do not apply.

18. A: None of their children will have sickle cell disease. With each pregnancy, there is a 50% probability of having a child with sickle cell trait and a 50% probability of having a child who is homozygous (AA).

19. D: The percentage of patients with dementia that are cared for in the home by family members is about 80%.

20. C: It is not a HIPAA violation to communicate with another provider via email.

21. A: Most people with high blood pressure have primary hypertension, meaning that there is no known cause. Secondary hypertension refers to high blood pressure with a known cause. Cocaine use, renal disease, and oral contraceptive use are all causes of secondary hypertension. Sepsis is associated with hypotension rather than hypertension.

22. D:Tamiflu (oseltamivir) is indicated for the treatment of uncomplicated illness due to influenza. To be effective, it must be started within 48 hours of onset of symptoms. Nausea, vomiting, and diarrhea are all common side effects of Tamiflu. Diarrhea is not a symptom routinely associated with influenza.

23. C: High fever for more than five days, cervical lymphadenopathy, nonexudative pharyngitis, red strawberry tongue, and maculopapular rash are hallmarks of Kawasaki disease. The fact that the illness did not respond to antibiotics and duration of fever makes the diagnosis of strep infection unlikely. This group of symptoms is not characteristic of either toxic epidermal necrolysis or juvenile rheumatoid arthritis.

24. B: A spouse is most likely to perpetrate abuse. The abuse may be either active or passive. Spouses feel most trapped in their situations of being caregivers and feel no hope of escape. A day-shift unrelated caregiver, by contrast, can leave and "decompress" after her shift.

25. C: The risk of suicide is over 60 times greater than normal in people with AIDS. In patients with chronic lung disease, the risk is 10 times greater. Comparatively speaking, diabetes and osteoporosis do not have high suicide rates.

26. D: Influenza virus is the most common cause of viral pneumonia in adults. Respiratory syncytial virus may be associated with pneumonia in children. *Haemophilus influenzae* is a bacterium, not a virus.

27. D: This patient has allergic conjunctivitis, which is associated with pruritus. Causes are allergens or environmental agents. Allergic conjunctivitis is not associated with increased intracranial pressure, fever, or myopia.

28. B: Acetaminophen is not an NSAID. Aspirin, indomethacin, and naproxen are all classified as NSAIDs. Acetaminophen reduces fever and pain has no anti-inflammatory properties.

29. C: Breast cancer causes the most cancer-related deaths in the 25 to 44 year age range. Lung cancer is the overall leading cause in patients of all ages. Hodgkin's disease occurs commonly in the 15- to 34-year age group and over age 60. The incidence of colon cancer peaks between 60 to 75 years of age. It is the second leading cause of cancer death in Western countries.

30. C: Iron-rich foods include leafy green vegetables, beans, egg yolks, fish, and poultry. Oranges are rich in vitamin C. Milk is rich in calcium and is typically not fortified with iron.

31. A: Herpangina is a viral illness caused by Coxsackie virus. Symptoms include fever, fussiness, throat pain, and drooling. In the early stages, vesicles appear on the tonsillar pillars. The vesicles subsequently ulcerate. Strep pharyngitis is uncommon at this age and is not associated with ulcerations. Gingivostomatitis, also viral, is associated with inflamed, bleeding gums, and mucosal ulcers over the anterior oral cavity. Epiglottitis is a severe, life-threatening bacterial infection associated with respiratory distress.

32. C: Norovirus (also called Norwalk-like virus) causes gastroenteritis. RSV, coronavirus, and rhinovirus have all been shown to cause bronchiolitis. Rhinovirus has recently been implicated in severe bronchiolitis illness. Human metapneumovirus is also an etiologic agent. In fact, the list of pathogens is growing.

33. C: People can have different concepts of time based on their cultures. Americans have more exacting standards for being on time. Hispanics (and others as well), often have a flexible interpretation of time and are more likely to be more approximate with their timelines. Providers should take cultural differences into account in healthcare settings.

34. A: Pneumovax is recommended for all patients 65 years and over. It can be administered with other vaccines but must be injected using a separate syringe at a different injection site. It should never be injected intradermally.

35.B: About one in three people over age 65 has some form of visual impairment. The number-one cause of loss of vision in this age group is age-related macular degeneration.

36. B: HSP is a type of vasculitis seen mostly in children. Patients with HSP often complain of abdominal pain. GI bleeding may also be present as well as joint pains. Patients should also be monitored for renal involvement by checking for hematuria. Purpura typically occurs on the buttocks and lower legs. Patients with HSP do not have thrombocytopenia, but may in fact have thrombocytosis.

37. D: A high-fiber diet is good advice for patients with GERD. Anticholinergic drugs are to be avoided, as they delay gastric emptying and thus would be counterproductive to the management of GERD. Excessive fat intake also delays gastric emptying, and it increases acid secretion in the stomach. Elevating the head of the bed helps prevent the flow of acid into the lower esophagus during sleep; however, the recommendation for elevation is 6 to 8 inches.

38. B: Bulk-forming laxatives such as psyllium (Metamucil) should be taken with a glass of water or other suitable liquid, immediately followed by a second glass. If not taken with enough fluid, it may cause choking or impaction of psyllium in the gastrointestinal tract. It is not necessary to take it with a calcium supplement.

39. C: The treatment of choice for an uncomplicated tooth abscess is penicillin VK. Erythromycin may also be used if the patient is allergic to penicillin. Extraction of the tooth is not necessary.

40. D: It is important maintain therapeutic communication with patients. Answers A, B, and C are nontherapeutic statements because of their defensive nature. Answer A has a punitive tone, implying a punishment of waiting an extra hour for attention. Answer B implies that the patient's problem is not worth the doctor's time. The correct answer, D, is therapeutic because it does not have a negative tone and it reinforces validation of the patient's feelings.

41. D: Umbilical hernias that are less than 2 cm in diameter will heal on their own. It is normal for an umbilical hernia to pouch out when intra-abdominal pressure increases, such as when the baby crying. This does not cause harm and will not cause enlargement of the abdominal wall defect that is present. Wrapping a band around the abdomen will not heal the hernia.

42. A: Perseveration is a repetitive, involuntary pathologic verbal or motor response to stimuli. It occurs in patients with organic mental disorders such as Alzheimer's disease and other forms of dementia. Repeating the same questions over and over is an example of perseveration. Contrivance refers to development of a clever scheme. By confabulating, a person makes up a plausible story or experience to compensate for memory lapses.

43. D: Symptoms of hypoglycemia include hunger, diaphoresis, light-headedness, tremors, nervousness, irritability, sleepiness, and confusion. Diplopia is not a symptom of low blood sugar.

44. B: Croup, also known as viral laryngotracheobronchitis, is associated with subglottic swelling, URI symptoms, and mild to moderate fever. The parainfluenza virus is a common cause. Routine croup is characterized by normal oxygen saturation and mild, if any, retractions. The hallmark is a barking or seal-like cough. On the other hand, fever of 104.5, tripod position, and drooling are signs of a life-threatening acute airway obstructive bacterial infection known as epiglottitis.

45. A: Breast cancer masses tend to be unilateral, firm, painless and irregular in shape. As the disease progresses, there may be redness and retraction of the nipple or the skin overlying the mass. A rubbery, smooth consistency is characteristic of a fibroadenoma, which is most common in women in their twenties and thirties.

46. A: Nursemaid's elbow (radial head subluxation) is common in toddlers, usually 1 to 4 years of age. As you take a history of the mechanism, it usually reveals that a parent suddenly pulled the child up by the arm as he started to fall. When the nursemaid's elbow is successfully reduced, the radial head relocates into its ligament. The clinician can usually feel a "pop" as it goes back into place.

47. B: Most anticoagulant treatment is directed toward a goal international normalized ratio (INR) of 2 to 3. An INR over 3 increases risk of bleeding. There are some autoimmune disorders associated with hypercoagulability necessitating an INR of 3 to 4.

48. B: Nicotine withdrawal is associated with bradycardia rather than tachycardia. Answers A, C, and D are all symptoms of nicotine withdrawal. Additional symptoms include poor concentration, irritability, depression, restlessness, and weight gain.

49. D: The penile foreskin serves a protective function for the glans penis. During the first 12 months of age, nearly all uncircumcised boys will have foreskin that tightly adheres to the glans. By 3 years of age, 90% will retract spontaneously. For some boys, it is normal to achieve retraction by age 5 or 6 years of age. Never forcibly retract the foreskin, as it is painful and may cause infection, phimosis, or paraphimosis.

50. C: Of all the choices given, only Hib (*Haemophilus influenzae*) vaccine is a conjugated vaccine. A conjugated vaccine is made from an altered organism that has been combined with a protein. Conjugation heightens the immune response to the vaccine.

51. C: Rotavirus has long been recognized as a cause of substantial morbidity in pediatric patients from infancy to age five years. An earlier version of the vaccine was taken off the market because of an associated incidence of intussusception, an obstructive condition in which one section of intestine "telescopes" into an adjacent section. Since the introduction of the current vaccine, intussusception rates have not increased beyond the expected range for this age group.

52. D: Antibodies to the killed influenza viruses used to prepare the vaccine form in approximately 2 weeks. The other answer choices are obviously incorrect.

53. B: Physical barriers are impediments that result from inadequate functioning of one or more systems of the body. These include vision, hearing, and mobility. In the case of this patient, his eyesight is impaired and he has limited mobility. Other barriers are psychological (such as emotional instability) and cognitive (such as dementia).

54. C: Frequent pacifier use is not associated with an increased risk of infant tooth decay. Decay may occur when an infant sleeps with a bottle of formula in his mouth and occurs regardless of the number of teeth present. Even babies who are exclusively breastfed can develop dental caries.

55. A: Reliable hearing screening results can be obtained as early as the newborn period.

56. B: Eye contact utilization varies from one culture to another. In some cultures, direct eye contact is considered rude, while in others, it is the desired norm. Observation of eye contact behaviors through experience working with different cultures can help you appreciate differences in eye contact customs.

57. D: When delegating a task to an unlicensed assistant, the nurse practitioner is responsible for providing ongoing supervision if the assistant needs help. In addition, the nurse practitioner is ultimately responsible for the appropriate completion of the task. An

unlicensed assistant unfamiliar with the task should not be called upon by another unlicensed assistant to complete an assignment.

58. B: Failure to monitor a patient is an example of medical negligence. Delegating routine tasks to a trained assistant, giving sound medical advice over the telephone, and referring a patient to a specialist are all appropriate actions.

59. B: Nurse practitioner scopes of practice do vary widely from state to state. Contrary to the statements in the answer choices, nurse practitioners may prescribe narcotics in most states and can also perform evaluations of psychosocial status.

60. A: Scabies is caused by the mite *Sarcoptes scabiei.* Mites are in the arachnid family and have eight legs. Insects have six. Ticks and protozoans are not etiologic factors in scabies infestation.

61. B: Rosacea is a chronic dermatosis. Characteristic features include facial redness, papules, and rhinophyma (hyperplasia of nasal tissue). It is commonly found on the cheeks, chin, forehead, and nose. Complications are dry eyes, deep painful facial nodules (pyoderma faciale), folliculitis, and blepharitis.

62. C: Approximately 30% of patients who have gallstones experience biliary colic, and about 10% will develop acute cholecystitis. Less common (< 1%) complications are gallbladder hydrops, small bowel obstruction, pancreatitis, and gallbladder perforation.

63. D: Because the lesion is localized, topical antifungal treatment is sufficient. In cases where lesions are generalized, oral antifungal therapy is appropriate and more practical. Topical corticosteroids, such as betamethasone, only suppress itching and inflammation. Topical diphenhydramine is not an antifungal medication, but rather an anti-itch product.

64. C: Over two-thirds of Bell's palsy patients recover completely and spontaneously. Approximately 15% have only mild sequelae.

65. A: Key components of overall management of osteoarthritis are nonpharmacological including exercise, physical therapy, thermal therapy, and weight loss if indicated. Joint replacement surgery and arthroscopy may eventually be needed, but not initially. Etanercept (Enbrel) is indicated for treatment of rheumatoid arthritis.

66. D: Hemoglobin A1c is typically measured every three to six months, depending on the desired tightness of glycemic control. Diabetics should also receive retinal exams at least once yearly to screen for retinopathy. In addition, urine should be tested for protein. If protein is negative, a screen for microalbuminuria would also be appropriate. Lipid measurement and control are routine in the management of Type 2 diabetes.

67. C: Basal cell carcinoma accounts for approximately 60% of primary skin cancers, while squamous cell carcinoma comprises 20%. Although most skin cancer deaths are from malignant melanoma, it is relatively rare and accounts for only 1% of skin cancers. Mycosis fungoides is a cutaneous T-cell lymphoma that initially appears in the skin but involves the whole reticuloendothelial system.

68. D: Developmental categories of Denver II are gross motor, fine motor, language, and personal/social. The test evaluates development in children from ages one month to six years.

69. C: Tobacco use in pregnancy is associated with numerous adverse outcomes. Maternal smoking accounts for over 20% of low-birth-weight infants. Other associated problems are placenta previa, preterm birth, placental abruption, and an increased risk of miscarriage.

70. C: Neural tube defects (NTDs) are congenital malformations caused by failure of neural tube closure during embryologic development. The neural tube forms the brain, spinal cord, and other central nervous system tissues. Folic acid protects against development of NTD. According to the Centers for Disease Control, all women who may potentially become pregnant should take folic acid daily.

71. A: Normal breast development may start as early as 8 years of age or as late as age 13 years. The girl in this clinical scenario is not, therefore, developing breasts prematurely and does not need medical evaluation.

72. C: Numerous medications are known to cause the side effect of peripheral edema. Rosiglitazone, an insulin sensitizer, can cause peripheral edema as in this patient. Neither SSRIs (Paxil and others) metformin, nor thiazide diuretics (hydrochlorothiazide) are associated with this side effect.

73. C: The majority of experts agree that routine preoperative electrocardiograms should be conducted on all men over age 45, patients with a history of heart disease, and patients with hypertension. Costochondritis is an inflammation of the anterior chest wall and is not associated with an abnormal ECG.

74. C: The patient in this clinical scenario is low risk. The incidence of an abnormal Pap test is low in women who have been screened at 65 years of age. According to the American Cancer Society, the recommendation for stopping is 70 years.

75. B: Of the choices given, only Pneumovax is appropriate. It is recommended for all persons over 65. FluMist is given to healthy patients under age 50. People born before 1957 are considered immune and do not need MMR. Hib vaccine is given to children under 6 years of age.

76. B: Only the 2-year-old may receive prophylaxis with Tamiflu. Oseltamivir (Tamiflu) is generally not recommended in children under 12 months of age.

77. C: Patients appreciate the opportunity to make choices from a list of viable options when they are available. Contrary to what many believe, patients often feel they have not received enough information rather than too much. Leaning toward patients has been shown to improve recall. Patients often do not understand or recall information, making it important to use techniques that help improve patient recall such as moving closer to the patient and increasing eye contact.

78. D: Of the choices given, obesity has a higher prevalence among Native Americans. Other conditions that are more prevalent in Native Americans when compared to other populations are diabetes, alcoholism, and suicide.

79. A: The principle of professional appearance is not one of the fundamental principles of professionalism. The true principles are as follows: primacy of patient welfare (serving the interest of the patient and not doing harm), patient autonomy (empowering patients to make informed treatment decisions), and social justice (eliminating discrimination in healthcare).

80. C: Disclosing this information would be a violation of patient confidentiality. The desire not to disclose protected information is the patient's prerogative, even if his wife asks for disclosure.

81. C: Family nurse practitioners often give anticipatory guidance to children and parents. Because children move from one developmental phase to another, parents need guidance on what to expect in certain areas of concern. Common areas for discussion for two-year-olds are growth and development, nutrition, emotional development, and safety. As children grow older, sports, exercise, sexual development, and warnings about drug abuse become important.

82. C: Rosacea is a chronic skin problem that is common in middle age. Most people with rosacea develop a cyclic pattern of disease. It may be confused with acne, but unlike acne, patients with rosacea do not develop comedones. Telangiectasia is common on the cheeks and nose with rosacea. The classic lupus malar rash is butterfly shaped and involves the cheeks and bridge of the nose. Seborrheic dermatitis appears on the face, upper chest, and any other areas of oily skin. There are often flaky, greasy white, or yellow scales present.

83. D: Temporomandibular dysfunction is a common cause of referred ear pain, making the other choices unlikely.

84. B: All of the choices given predispose patients to recurrent sinus infections. However, allergic rhinitis is the most common one of those listed. Allergic rhinitis is seen in approximately 60% of patients with recurrent sinusitis.

85. A: This patient is exhibiting body language that poses a barrier to communication with the provider by him appearing disinterested. Gestures are performed with hands or with the head as in nodding in agreement or waving hands to mimic an activity. Facial expressions show emotions such as happiness or fear. Empathy is not a type of nonverbal communication.

86. D: It is sometimes necessary to use an interpreter in a clinical setting. The interpreter should be medically trained. The provider should address the patient directly, as if the interpreter was not there. Use a normal voice volume and try to employ simple language, expressing one concept at a time. Place chairs in a triangular configuration and face the patient while speaking.

87. C: All healthcare professionals should have a commitment to quality of care. In this scenario, the nurse practitioner should act in the best interest of the patient. The correct response is to call the error to the physician's attention in a professional manner. It is unprofessional to tell a patient that a physician is incompetent.

88. A: Drug-seeking patients often claim "allergies" to various pain medications and claim that only one specific narcotic works for their pain. In addition, drug seekers usually hop

from one doctor to another to get the drugs they want. The term "drug seeker" applies to a person who is trying to obtain narcotics. The term is not usually used to refer to patients who want antibiotics.

89. D: This patient has bacterial vaginosis. A KOH prep characteristically reveals a fishy odor and clue cells. The treatment is metronidazole. Doxycycline is used to treat Chlamydia. Terconazole is used to treat vaginal candidiasis and ceftriaxone is used to treat gonococcal infections.

90. A: Fifth disease is primarily a disease of children. It produces the so-called slapped cheek rash and is caused by parvovirus B19. The other answer choices are incorrect.

91. D: Accutane (an acne drug) is a known teratogen that belongs to pregnancy category X. In fact, it is best not taken by women of childbearing age unless acne is extremely severe and unresponsive to other therapies. It is associated with a high potential for fetal injury. Healthcare providers perform a pregnancy test on the patient before starting Accutane and will likely continue doing pregnancy tests monthly prior to prescription renewal.

92. B: By identifying a problem, you are employing the process of assessment. Planning involves the process of determining an action plan. Implementation carries out the plan, and evaluation involves examining and appraising the plan of action.

93. C: Interpersonal conflict exists between one person and another, whereas intrapersonal conflict is an internal conflict involving only one person.

94. A: A diversion program is a voluntary alternative to disciplinary action by attending group sessions such as Narcotics Anonymous, Alcoholics Anonymous, and counseling. The person also voluntarily submits urine for periodic drug testing. Some facilities allow diversion program nurses to work in their units under specific guidelines. Most states allow petitions to the board for full licensure reinstatement after 12 to 24 months by showing proof of full compliance with the program and by showing ability to perform in the workplace.

95. D: Licensure by examination is required when a state does not grant licensure by reciprocity and a candidate must pass an examination in that state. A temporary license allows a nurse to practice while the license is pending. Licensure by waiver occurs if the candidate meets or exceeds some licensure requirements. These requirements can be waived, but the nurse must be able to demonstrate other requirements.

96. C: Unlicensed assistive personnel should never perform tasks that require complex problem-solving skills. They may perform tasks with a low risk of harming the patient and tasks that are highly likely to result in positive outcomes.

97. D: While surgically removing the wrong body part is an egregious error, it does not involve a medication-related error.

98. B: A duty to patients supersedes merely following doctor's orders. Acting as a patient advocate is a vital nursing function. In fact, a nurse has a duty to report medical care that could jeopardize patient care.

99. A: This process is known as risk management. Quality assurance is an evaluation of medical services, their results, and how they compare to the accepted standards. Patient rights are a form of nursing intervention involving healthcare rights.

100. D: If you do not actually witness an event such as a fall, you cannot speculate on how it happened. You must document things as you see them when you initially encounter the situation. In this case, the only thing you can accurately state is that you found the patient lying on the floor face-down when you entered the area.

101. A: Nurse practice acts are established by state legislatures to regulate nursing practice in each state. The acts vary somewhat from state to state. Each nurse is responsible for knowing the provisions for the state in which he or she works. Nurse practice acts *do* set educational requirements. Answer C defines an ethics committee rather than a nurse practice act.

102. C: If a nurse walks out on his/her job as in this case because of understaffing, he or she could be charged with abandonment. Fraud involves deception that produces illegal personal gain. Defamation is a false statement that damages a person's reputation. Collective bargaining is a process whereby management and labor representatives negotiate working conditions and wages.

103. C: Answer choices A, B, and D are all correct. The incident report form should not be copied nor placed in the patient's record.

104. A: You should strongly suspect gram-negative organisms as the cause of conjunctivitis in contact lens wearers. Topical gentamicin or tobramycin would therefore be a good choice for treatment. In people who do not wear contact lenses, bacterial conjunctivitis is most commonly caused by either *Staphylococcus aureus* or *Streptococcus pneumoniae*.

105. B: GER is a common cause of vomiting in infants. It may also be associated with episodes of recurrent wheezing. This patient is too old to be presenting with pyloric stenosis, which typically manifests itself with recurrent vomiting within three to five weeks after birth and is rare in babies over three months of age. Viral gastroenteritis is self-limited and does not last two months. Reactive airway disease is associated with wheezing but not with vomiting.

106. B: To determine BMI, divide the patient's weight in kilograms by their height in meters squared. A BMI greater than 25 is overweight. If the BMI is more than 30, the patient is considered obese. Morbidly obese patients have BMIs over 35.

107. D: An estimated 65% of Americans are overweight and about 35% are obese.

108. C: The patient in this clinical scenario has post-streptococcal glomerulonephritis (PSGN). The source of the strep infection was the impetigo. Children often present with periorbital edema because of a loss of protein in the urine. A diagnosis of UTI is not likely, given the symptoms of painless hematuria and edema. Painless hematuria requires investigation. Kidney stones are associated with intermittent severe colicky pain.

109. C: A fluoroquinolone such as levofloxacin is a good choice of antibiotic considering there was treatment failure with first-line drugs. First-generation cephalosporins and

erythromycin are not recommended because they do not provide adequate coverage of major pathogens. In addition, clarithromycin may not provide coverage for resistant *Streptococcus pneumoniae.*

110. A: Of the choices given, an MRI is the best choice. A herniated disk will not show up on a plain radiograph. Bend-over tests screen for scoliosis. Loss of range of motion is nonspecific.

111. D: Placing allergen-blocking covers on the mattress and pillows are a good way to decrease asthma triggers. Frequent vacuuming and use of ceiling fans actually help spread allergen particles into the air. Home humidity levels should ideally be less than 50%.

112. A: Tricyclic antidepressants such as amitriptyline and SSRIs such as citalopram are often associated with sexual dysfunction. Of the choices given, bupropion is least likely to cause sexual side effects.

113. C: This patient is showing signs and symptoms of rheumatoid arthritis: proximal interphalangeal joint involvement of the hands, symmetrical swelling, fatigue, and prolonged morning stiffness. Symptoms of osteoarthritis usually develop gradually. Joints of the hips, back, base of the thumb and neck are often affected in osteoarthritis. Psoriatic arthritis occurs in patients who have psoriasis. In this type of arthritis, joints are less symmetrically involved. Gout most often involves the joints of the feet.

114. D: The patient in this scenario has symptoms of acute glaucoma. This is a medical emergency. The only correct answer is to refer the patient immediately to an ophthalmologist.

115. C: All household and close contacts should be treated with azithromycin or clarithromycin, which each have fewer side effects and are associated with better patient compliance with once-daily dosing. The medication is taken by close contacts and household members regardless of immunization status. This helps limit the transmission of infection to others.

116. B: This clinical scenario raises strong suspicion for cystic fibrosis. CF is more common in Caucasians and is associated with frequent respiratory infections and digestive problems such as diarrhea and greasy stools (high fat content). These finding are not characteristic of either thyroid disorders or tuberculosis. Performing a sweat chloride test will aid in the diagnosis of CF.

117. D: A newborn infant exhibits the Moro reflex in response to a loud noise such as a hand clap. This reflex is also known as the startle reflex. Stimulation of the perioral area elicits the rooting reflex. The tonic neck reflex occurs when you turn the newborn's head to one side and he assumes a "fencing posture."

118. D: A short-acting beta-2 agonist, such as albuterol or levalbuterol, is appropriate for use as a rescue medication. Corticosteroid inhalers, leukotriene inhibitors, and anti-allergic medications are useful for long-term control.

119. C: An initial symptom of tuberculosis is a mild cough productive of nonbloody mucoid sputum. Bloody sputum production, chest pain, and breathing difficulty are all late symptoms.

120. A: The infant has a candida diaper rash, which is usually treated with nystatin cream. The use of talcum powder is no longer recommended due to the risk of aspiration of particles by the infant and because it was not shown to be effective in decreasing moisture in the diaper area. Oral fluconazole is not first-line treatment for cutaneous candidiasis. Mupirocin is useful in the treatment of localized bacterial skin infections.

121. C: Mucoceles are usually caused by trauma to the inner lining of the lip. They rupture easily and spontaneously. Most patients with mucoceles are under age 20 years. Unroofing or aspirating the lesion is associated with recurrences. If the patient has frequent recurrences, refer them to an oral surgeon.

122. B: Enuresis is more common in boys than girls. UTI is not a common cause of nocturnal enuresis. A renal ultrasound is usually not necessary. Imipramine has a success rate of less than 50%.

123. C: This child most likely has a viral URI. Allergic rhinitis and nasal foreign bodies are not associated with fever. In addition, nasal foreign bodies cause unilateral nasal discharge. The yellow color of the mucus is not significant. Symptoms of four days' duration are highly unlikely to be caused by sinusitis, which is uncommon at this age anyway.

124. B: A chest x-ray is recommended for asymptomatic patients with a positive PPD to rule out the slight possibility of an active TB infection. Treatment with INH decreases the progression of latent TB to active TB infection. Nine months is the optimal duration of treatment. A sputum culture is done if there are findings of old TB on chest x-ray.

125. C: Children with a cleft palate are at increased risk for recurrent otitis media. Children with clefts are more likely to develop fluid behind the tympanic membrane. Usually the fluid drains through the Eustachian tube, but the tube is often distorted by the cleft and interferes with proper drainage. During surgical repair of the cleft, surgeons usually insert ventilator tubes in the eardrum to allow fluid to drain.

126. B: Colic, sudden infant death syndrome (SIDS), and wheezing are all associated with cigarette smoke exposure. Bacterial conjunctivitis is not associated with exposure to smoking.

127. B: About 50% of people who travel abroad become ill while traveling. The most common illness is traveler's diarrhea. The other illnesses listed as answer choices are less frequent.

128. C: Of all the choices given, women are most likely to be interested in using alternative medicine therapies.

129. A: The mainstay of treatment for viral diarrhea in children is to maintain adequate hydration. If the child with diarrhea is not vomiting, there is no need to stop feeding solid foods. Antidiarrheal and antispasmodic medications are not recommended for children.

130. C: Intermittent claudication is an aching, cramping, or burning in the legs due to poor circulation in the arteries. It often occurs with walking and disappears with rest. It is not normal and can be due to atherosclerosis or vasospasm. Restless legs syndrome is a neurologic disorder associated with an unpleasant sensation in the legs and with a compulsion to move the legs. Multiple sclerosis is also a neurologic disorder.

131. C: The ESR is an acute phase reactant. An elevated ESR is indicative of inflammation, but it is not specific for any disorder. In performing the test, red blood cells are allowed to settle in a tube of unclotted blood. At the end of one hour, the distance the cells have fallen is measured. Inflammation produces a change in blood proteins, causing red blood cells to aggregate and become heavier than normal and therefore take longer to form sediment at the bottom of the tube.

132. A: As in this case, an infant given free water is at risk for developing hyponatremia. Low levels of sodium are associated with seizures. Infants who need hydration should be given an oral electrolyte solution or intravenous fluids rather than plain water.

133. A: The Adams forward bend test is used to screen for scoliosis. The test is performed by asking the patient to bend forward 90 degrees at the waist, as if to touch his toes. The examiner looks for asymmetry of the trunk (an asymmetric thoracic prominence on one side). The test has its limitations in that it cannot detect the exact severity of scoliosis, nor can it detect lower spine curvatures.

134. C: Contributory negligence occurs when the patient contributes to his own negative outcome.

135. B: To calculate BMI, divide the weight in kilograms by the height in meters squared. In this example, BMI = 64 divided by (1.6 x 1.6) = 64/2.54 = 25.

136. D: A child subsisting on a diet of mostly whole milk is at risk for developing iron deficiency anemia. Whole milk is not iron fortified. Because he is not eating any solid foods, there are no other sources of iron in his diet.

137. B: The patient in this clinical scenario has a prolapsed uterus. The uterus is the only organ that can fall into the vagina. Depending on duration and severity, the uterus can become ulcerated and result in bleeding. This is often the result of child bearing and weakening of the pelvic tissues as a woman ages. It is common for urinary incontinence to exist in these cases.

138. A: Retinal detachment is typically not associated with eye pain. The patient complains of seeing floaters, flashes of light, and loss of the central portion of vision.

139. B: Direct inguinal hernias are generally acquired due to heavy lifting, straining, or coughing. Indirect inguinal hernias, hiatal hernias in children, and umbilical hernias in infants are congenital.

140. C: Bedsores have rating stages depending on the amount of damage done to the body. A stage 1 bedsore consists of a well-defined area of persistent redness without skin breakdown or pain. Bedsores frequently form in the sacral area and other areas of high

friction. Cellulitis is a skin infection characterized by redness, tenderness, warmth, and induration over the involved area. Abscesses are infections that contain pus.

141. D: A nurse can be sued for malpractice for various reasons including failure to report a change in a patient's condition, failure to answer calls from a patient, neglecting to monitor a patient, administering the wrong medication, and administering a treatment not ordered by the physician. All nurses should maintain continuing education requirements, but failing to do so is not grounds for a malpractice suit.

142. B: This patient has otitis externa. Topical treatment with combination antibiotic and corticosteroid drops has been shown to be very effective. Because the inflammation is localized, systemic antibiotics are rarely indicated. Antipyrine/benzocaine drops are ineffective. Ibuprofen may help with pain, but by itself, it is not the best answer.

143. D: The developmental milestones are closest to those of a 9-month-old. Infants that are 8 to 10 months old are able to use a pincer grasp, pull up to stand, and walk holding onto furniture, and recognize the word "no."

144. B: Breast development in adolescent boys can be very distressing. These patients are often teased at school. However, it is a temporary and benign condition due to hormonal imbalances of estrogen and testosterone during puberty. It affects 40 to 60% of male teens. No treatment, workups, or referrals are needed.

145. C: Routine nosebleeds often originate from Kiesselbach's plexus over the anterior nasal septum. To stop a nosebleed, pinch the nostrils shut and apply continuous pressure for 10 minutes. Applying pressure to the nasal bridge, tilting the head back, and applying ice packs to the forehead are common mistakes people make when treating nosebleeds.

146. A: Venous stasis dermatitis is an inflammatory skin disease that occurs in the lower extremities of middle-aged and elderly patients. It is caused by venous insufficiency that occurs when venous valves become incompetent.

147. C: Peak flow is a useful measure of asthma control. Peak flow meters measure the air flow out of the lungs as a patient blows forcefully into the device. Measurements between 80 to 100% of personal best are in the green zone, indicating good control. Measurements at 50 to 79% are in the yellow zone, a caution indicating some loss of asthma control. Adjustments may need to be made with medications. The red zone is a reading less than 50% of personal best and indicates a need for immediate medical attention.

148. D: The recommended ratio of chest compressions to breaths in adult CPR is 30:2. The same ratio applies to children and older infants.

149. B: Ciprofloxacin may be used safely and effectively for prophylaxis of traveler's diarrhea. Increased resistance has limited the effectiveness of trimethoprim-sulfa and doxycycline.

150. B: The treatment of choice for gonococcal cervicitis is intramuscular ceftriaxone.